HOW TO USE THIS BOOK

Healthy, Happy YOU makes self-improvement bite-sized.
Give the book just one minute of your day, every day,
and it will give you simple micro-actions you can do
for a healthier, happier you.

When you've completed a micro-action, tick it off in the
square provided at the top of the page. You'll find space
on every page to write down your thoughts and note
down your achievements. There are also "Reflect and
Renew" sections throughout.

What is a micro-action?
A micro-action is small, simple, and achievable in a
normal day. For anyone. "Meditate for twenty minutes"
isn't a micro-action, but "sit quietly for two minutes" is.
"Run a marathon" isn't a micro-action, but "take the
stairs" is. Simple, but they make all the difference.

MICRO-ACTION CATEGORIES

Each micro-action falls under one of these four categories:

FOOD: Food is such an integral part of how you live that small, simple changes in how you eat can add years to your life. "Food" micro-actions are not only about what you eat but how, when, how much, and with whom. "Stop eating chocolate" is not a micro-action. "Snack on a veggie" is.

MIND: The mind determines who you are and how you act. But it isn't set in stone – it can be trained. "Mind" micro-actions tackle mindfulness (being present in the moment), productivity, and organization (making sense of the world around us). "Clean the house" is not a micro-action. "Organize a kitchen cabinet" is.

MOVE: "Move" micro-actions are about everyday movement – small, easy micro-actions that you can incorporate into your daily routine. "Sign up for a triathlon" is not a micro-action. "Do two minutes of heel kicks" is.

LOVE: Don't be fooled by the title – it's not about romance. "Love" micro-actions are about your relationship with yourself and with others. Here, micro-actions really matter. Treating someone well triggers a positive reaction in that person, which triggers a positive reaction in you, too. "Make a new friend" is not a micro-action. "Reach out to someone" is.

healthy,
happy
YOU

365 DAILY MICRO-ACTIONS
FOR LASTING CHANGE

THE EXPERIMENT

NEW YORK

SMALL THINGS MATTER

We all have it in us to live a healthy, happy life!
Yet self-improvement can be difficult, and knowing
what to do on a day-to-day basis is not always
obvious or intuitive.

**Your life is the sum of the small micro-actions
you do every day, and every choice you make
is significant.**

This book will empower you to make change
happen – one micro-action at a time.

Because the small things matter.

HOW DO I START?

There are 365 micro-actions in this book: one for each day of the year. We suggest you start with number 1, then after the first few you can either follow the daily order or jump around to mix things up – it's completely up to you!

HOW DO I MAKE THE MOST OF IT?

• **Take your time** – Change works most effectively in small steps, so don't try to overachieve. Take your time, and reflect on each micro-action.

• **Be open** – Be open to different micro-actions, but if the micro-action is just not for you, simply turn to a different page and perhaps come back to it another day.

• **Repeat micro-actions** – The key to creating lasting change is to form new habits. Having a habit means your brain does it on autopilot, and it can last you a lifetime. We call the actions you're repeating to form a habit "Keep It Up" actions. Many habits can be formed in around twenty-eight days, so use the "Reflect and Renew" pages to record and follow up on them.

• **Make it your own** – We're all different, so make this book work for you. Write in it. Doodle in it. Carry it around as a companion. Flip through the pages. Skip micro-actions. Redo micro-actions. Do it alone, or with your loved ones.

Get ready to start living a healthier, happier life, for you.

THE BACK STORY

Healthy, Happy YOU was born out of an app called YOU-app. We at YOU-app have always been passionate about health and personal change, and the road here has been an interesting one.

We know that change is hard for most people.
We all make big resolutions and struggle to fulfill them. In fact, 9 out of 10 fail, resulting in us feeling worse about ourselves.

We've been there. We've struggled with the same issues as most people – finding that elusive "work-life balance," feeding your body right, cultivating a healthy self-image, and not getting bogged down in the stresses of everyday life.

We wanted a simpler approach. We started working on micro-actions because science – as well as our own experiences – has proved it's the small changes that truly make a difference. Micro-actions build the habit of success, and behaving just a bit differently inspires more awareness and personal progress.

And so, YOU-app was born. The movement of YOU is about the power of small changes to have a real impact on your life. We want to bring a sound, fresh voice to the diet-crazy, transformation-obsessed world of self-improvement.

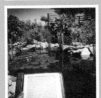

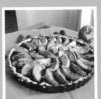

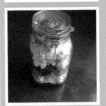
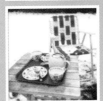

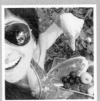
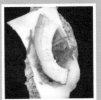

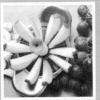

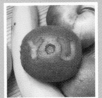

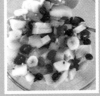
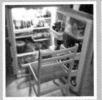

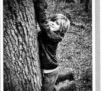
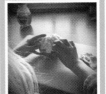

WHO WE ARE

YOU is a team effort. The team consists of designers, developers, micro-action creators, the marketing team, and the brilliantly warm and supportive YOU community.

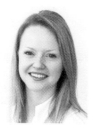

Former management consultant turned eager entrepreneur, **Nora Rosendahl** is the editorial engine behind the YOU micro-actions. Engineer by background and with years of experience solving tough business problems for some of the world's largest companies, she's often the odd one out in the health start-up scene. A meditative weekend spent in self-reflection changed the course of her career, and Nora now combines creative writing, empathetic community management, and hardcore number crunching on a daily basis for YOU.

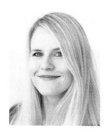

Engineer by background, entrepreneur through passion, and musician at heart, **Nelli Lähteenmäki** is a true people connector. An interest in sales took her to San Francisco, a passion for growth entrepreneurship made her stay, and a longing to build a health start-up made her return to Finland and start the journey that eventually led to YOU. A bundle of positive energy and with a network to die for, Nelli can navigate any start-up scene like a lioness on the savanna plains.

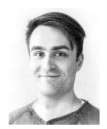

With a determined, thoughtful and decisive touch, **Aleksi Hoffman** steers the direction of the YOU product. He has a background in engineering and bioelectronics, so can be trusted to code anything from health care IT to IPTV systems. A passion for personal behavior change, a visual eye to match any professional designer, a heart of gold, and a perfect overhead squatting technique make Aleksi a solid rock to lean on.

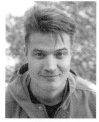

The designing duo other teams would kill for, **Jaakko Hyvärinen** and **Toni Sallinen** are the powerhouse behind the YOU brand and visual identity. With a creative touch, crazy humor, and a human-centric approach, they carefully craft the YOU we know and love.

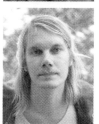

And it's not just us, we've made some good company along the way. We've had creative writing assistance from Isabel Hayman-Brown and Tiina Liukkonen, and we've enlisted the help of category-specific experts, such as Jamie Oliver and Caroline Arnold. You can find out more about all of our guest contributors on the next few pages.

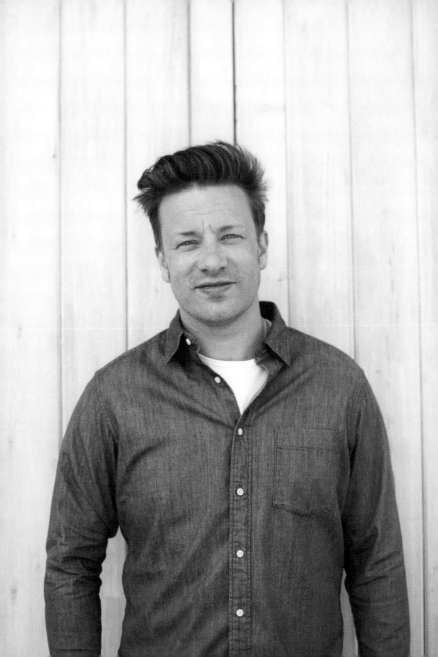

CONTRIBUTOR BIOGRAPHIES

Jamie Oliver (Food)

Jamie's micro-actions exist to help everyone eat better and have a healthier relationship with food, one step at a time. After refocusing on his own health over the last two years, YOU-app has provided a powerful platform for Jamie to offer up his in-depth food knowledge, as well as tips he learned while earning a recent qualification in nutrition. Jamie is a global phenomenon in food and food campaigning. Over a sixteen-year television and publishing career, he has inspired millions of people to enjoy cooking from scratch and eat fresh, delicious food.

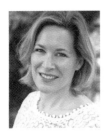

Caroline Arnold (Mind)

Caroline is the author of *Small Move, Big Change: Using Microresolutions to Transform Your Life Permanently*. As well as being an advisor for the YOU-app and an international speaker on how to exploit the dynamics of personal change to achieve permanent self-improvement, Caroline is also a managing director at Goldman Sachs in New York.

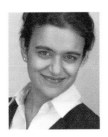

Dr. Tara Swart (Mind)

Dr. Swart is an Oxford-trained medical doctor who worked in psychiatry for seven years, has a PhD in neuroscience, and started a brain-based leadership consultancy in 2008. She is the author of two books, as well as a global speaker on sustainable behavior change and resilience.

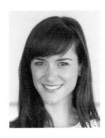

Darya Rose (Food)

Darya is the author of *Foodist* and creator of Summer Tomato, one of TIME's 50 Best Websites. She received her PhD in neuroscience from the University of California, San Francisco, and her bachelor's degree in molecular and cell biology from the University of California, Berkeley. Darya spends most of her time thinking and writing about food, health, and science.

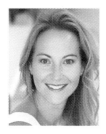

Dani Stevens (Move)
Dani believes in starting small but dreaming big. In her ten-year journey to fitness and well-being, she has lost close to 220 pounds over the course of four pregnancies. A busy mom, she proves that you don't need an army of fitness trainers and private chefs to turn the dream of enjoying a healthy lifestyle into reality. As a fitness-food motivator, DaniStevens.com has a community of over 200,000 people across the globe.

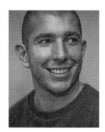

Jamie Sawyer (Move)
Jamie is one of the UK's leading strength and conditioning coaches and is also a personal trainer. His experience has taken him from working with elite athletes to Hollywood A-listers. Jamie uses his knowledge of sports science to create custom training, nutrition, and lifestyle regimes.

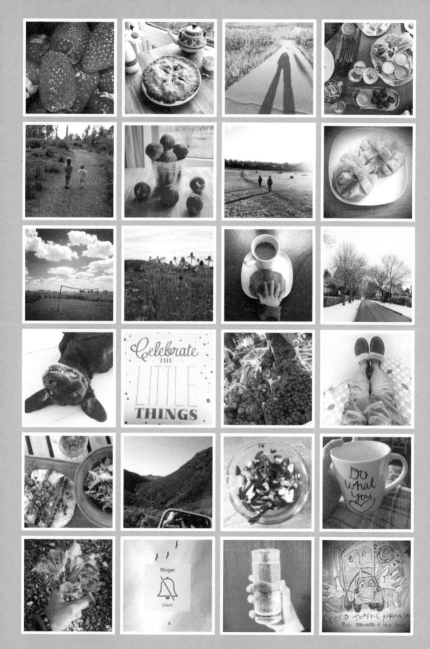

1. **USING THIS BOOK**

Making the decision to live happily and healthily is the crucial first step toward changing your life for the better.

Use *Healthy, Happy YOU* in the way that suits you best – on your nightstand as a daily journal to record your micro-actions and thoughts; as a coffee-table book to give you occasional inspiration; or carry it around with you to reach for when you have a spare minute. So today, simply reflect on how best to make time for you every day and on what you hope to achieve from this book.

....

....

....

....

....

....

....

2. **THANK A PERSON WHO MAKES YOU HAPPY**

Having positive people around you gives you energy
and a more positive outlook on life. Take a moment to reflect on
someone you love who's a positive force in your life.
How could you show your thanks to them?

3. **LET'S GET PHYSICAL**

You don't have to climb mountains, pound treadmills, or
lift weights to get active. Research shows that just working
small, extra movement into your day has amazing health
benefits. Make a regular journey more physical – park at
the far end of the parking lot or climb the stairs instead of
using the escalator. Whatever it is, no matter how big
or small, just get moving more. **Jamie S**

4. **TAKE A MOMENT**

Take a moment without any disturbances to simply observe
your surroundings. When life feels busy we often forget to
take the "me time" that our minds need to relax, refresh, and
regroup. Do you regularly take time during the day to pause?
Observe your surroundings for five minutes.

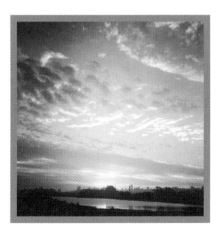

5. **FILL YOUR FRUIT BOWL**

Today, stock up your fruit bowl, and if you don't have one –
get one! I like to think of fruit as nature's candy store – it's
delicious, pretty much the simplest snack there is, and of
course it's all packed with different and wonderful vitamins,
minerals, and nutrients. To see snacking on fruit as a pleasure,
and not a chore, just fill your fruit bowl with lots of lovely,
colorful, seasonal choices. **Jamie**

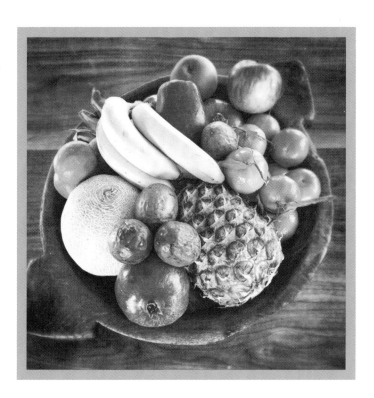

6. **YOUR COMMANDMENTS**

Why not devise some personal commandments?
Today, take a moment to think about what's important
to you and create three personal commandments –
for example, "Keep a positive outlook" or "Put family first."

Record them here:

....

....

....

....

....

....

7. **TAKE CARE OF YOURSELF**

Neglecting personal needs can impact your physical and
mental well-being, and putting off scheduling appointments
creates low-level anxiety that can dampen your productivity.
Today, schedule an appointment with a doctor, dentist,
accountant, or neglected friend. You'll feel more relaxed
immediately and it only takes a phone call. **Caroline**

8. **ENJOY THE WEATHER**

All weather is beautiful in its own right. Today,
take a few minutes and enjoy the weather outside,
whether it's rainy, sunny, or overcast. How will you
make the most of the weather?

9. HUMBLE H$_2$O

Being hydrated is super important as it means everything in our bodies works better – especially our brains, which are more than 70 percent water. Try swapping juice and soda for H$_2$O today. The cheapest way to hydrate is to turn on the tap. Water doesn't have to be boring: get creative with natural flavor combos. Think zingy citrus slices, cucumber ribbons, fresh mint or basil leaves, juicy berries, or fresh ginger. **Jamie**

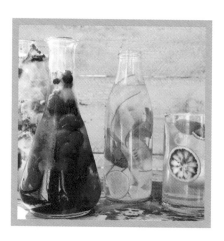

10. **PICK A NEW HABIT**

Whether it's brushing your teeth, washing your hair or putting on your makeup, habits constitute 40 percent of what you do every day. They're crucial to help rest the mind. Creating a new habit has the power to improve your health, appearance, productivity, relationships, and work life. And the magic of a habit is that once it's been established, it will support you for life. Decide on one micro-action you will make into a habit. Flip through the book to get inspiration on what your next new habit could be.

....

....

11. **MAKE YOURSELF SMILE**

How are you putting a smile on your own face today? Research shows that the mere act of smiling will actually make you feel happier! Do it early, and your smile can spread the mood to other people throughout the day.

12. **WORK IT IN TO WORK IT OUT**

Simply planning to exercise makes a big difference to whether you actually do it. Commit to a simple exercise routine for next week. Book it, call someone up to arrange a session, write it down – however simple it is, planning it will help you to make it happen. For an extra boost, lay out your gear the night before. **Jamie S**

13. **A QUICK FIX**

Today, fix something in ten minutes or less. Change a light bulb, sew a button on a shirt, install fresh batteries in a device, fertilize a plant. Repair just one thing. These tasks may not be critical, but completing one will make you feel back on top of things. **Caroline**

14. **PRACTICE MINDFUL EATING**

Eating better is not only about *what* you eat but *how*,
so try to practice mindful eating. Think about what you're
eating and why. At your next meal, take a moment to
appreciate the sensations. **Darya**

15. **PAY SOMEONE A COMPLIMENT**

Giving and receiving praise increases goodwill and lifts moods
in both the giver and receiver. Making someone feel good is
likely to make you feel good, too, putting a spring in your step.
Today, be mindful and vocal about the contributions and
positive attributes of others, and feel the boost. **Caroline**

16. **A HABIT TO HANG ON TO**

Here's a crazy fact – we make more than 200 decisions about food and drinks every day and, out of those, we are aware of fewer than 15 of them. Today, identify a good eating habit that you want to keep. Becoming a bit more aware of the choices you make when it comes to food is the first step to improving your overall health. **Jamie**

17. **UNSUBSCRIBE**

Is your inbox inundated with promotions and newsletters? Today, unsubscribe from unnecessary emails. See how many mailing lists you can remove yourself from in five minutes. Searching for the word "unsubscribe" in your inbox can help you target unwanted subscriptions. **Caroline**

18. **WRITE A SHOPPING LIST**

Sounds simple, doesn't it? But whether scribbled on the back of an envelope, keyed into your phone, or written in a cute little notebook, a shopping list could save you money and means you're less likely to impulse buy – which in turn can often mean spending too much money, buying food you don't need, and ending up with food waste. Follow this simple step and take a few minutes to write a shopping list to avoid that impulse-buy cycle. **Jamie**

19. TWO-MINUTE WORKOUT: STEP IT UP

Moving your body doesn't have to be hard – we have endless possibilities around us to add a bit of extra movement to the day, we just need to notice them. For example, use the stairs and steps around you. Two minutes spent walking up and down those will work up a real sweat. **Dani**

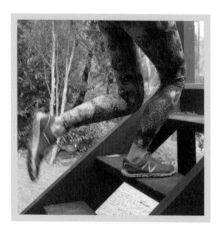

20. **MAKE A CONNECTION**

Happiness may seem like a fluffy, subjective topic, but extensive research on the science of happiness has shown that there are ten main factors that drive it. One of them is connecting to other people. Pick up the phone, send a postcard, order some flowers – connect to someone today.

21. **TAKE A REAL BREATH**

Our breathing is often too shallow. Try diaphragmatic breathing – it activates the lower parts of the lungs, which are seven times more efficient at helping our cells get in the good stuff (oxygen) and get rid of waste (carbon dioxide). This kind of breathing also has lots of other benefits, including calming us down and improving stress management, digestion, and blood pressure. Try it out. Place one hand on your chest and the other on your belly. Breathe in through your nose for three seconds, hold for three seconds, then exhale through your mouth for five seconds. Throughout the breathing, only the hand on your belly should move. **Jamie S**

22. **MAKE A DAILY ROUTINE INCONVENIENT**

If you build movement into your daily routine, you will ensure that you move more throughout the day – and it really adds up over time. Use a small glass so you have to get up to refill it with water more frequently, move the trash can to a different place, park at the far end of the parking lot, or walk the longer way round. **Jamie S**

23. **HOME EXERCISE**

We often think that being active involves spending hours at the gym, but you can achieve a healthy lifestyle much more simply. Add small micro-movements into your day. Get up and do squats over a chair, run up and down some stairs, take a walk around the house, or do some work in the garden to get that blood flowing. **Dani**

24. **A CULTURAL MICRO-EXPERIENCE**

Did you know that cultural activities improve the bond
between the two halves of your brain? Anything counts –
from reading a novel to attending an opera or going to
the theater, from visiting a gallery to writing a poem
or story, or even doodling. **Tara**

Try it here:

FOOD

25. A FAMILY MEAL

Sharing scrumptious food with the people you love is one of life's great pleasures. Take the time to enjoy a home-cooked family meal today or this week. Gather your loved ones around one table – whether that's your partner, a family spanning generations, or the bunch of friends you live with – and enjoy some tasty homemade grub. **Jamie**

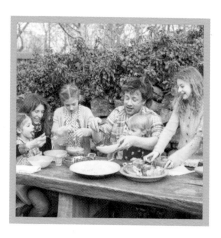

26. **JUST FEEL IT**

Notice how you are feeling today. Blue? Excited about the week to come? Nervous, happy, or hopeful? Write down a few thoughts and, if you're feeling negative, just let it go.

27. **TAKE STOCK**

Devote a bit of time today to take stock of the contents of
your fridge. I bet it gets to a certain point every so often when
your fridge – like mine – has been totally neglected. So dig
through and pull out all those half-used, leftover, and past-
their-prime items. Use them up – turn them into meals, freeze
them, or simply move them to the front of the fridge
so they're not forgotten. **Jamie**

28. **OFF WITH DIGITAL ALERTS**

It's hard to make progress on priorities when a beep, buzz, or
notification alert interrupts you every thirty seconds. This digital
chain-jerking can be a real drag on productivity. Turn off one or
more alerts today to regain some focus. **Caroline**

29. FIND MICRO-MAGIC IN YOUR DAY

Remember when you were a kid and everything around you had the potential to generate wonder and awe? Find some magic again today, be it in the sound of the rain, looking up at the moon, discovering something in nature, the laughter of a loved one, or a quiet moment alone.

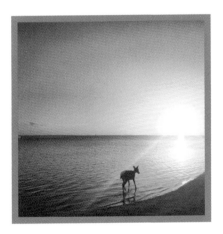

30.
REFLECT
AND
RENEW

As mentioned in the introduction, the most effective way to create lasting change is to create new habits. Many habits can be formed in around twenty-eight days.

Write down a few notes and feelings from the past weeks.

Do you have a favorite micro-action so far?

Now's the best time to pick one and make it your Keep It Up action for the month to come.

FOOD

31. **EAT GREEN**

Today is a simple one – eat something green. We all know that green stuff is good for us. Spinach might not make us Popeye-strong but it's loaded with vitamin A, which helps us see properly, especially in the dark. Greens like broccoli, peas, kale, and cabbage are packed with vitamin C, which our bodies need for pretty much anything and everything. Embrace those greens in a meal today! **Jamie**

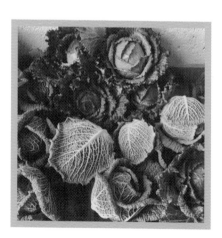

32. **TACKLE ONE BAD EATING HABIT**

We've all got bad habits that catch up with us, so today is
time to fess up. Identify one bad eating habit and tackle it,
proactively making a healthier choice instead. You could swap
a soda for naturally flavored water, eat rather than skip
breakfast, swap that 4 PM sugar fix for something wholesome,
or just be a bit more mindful about your portion control. **Jamie**

33. **LISTEN TO A POWERFUL SONG**

Music can make us do and feel all sorts of things:
feel better, run faster, smile, cry, or recall a memory.
So listen to a song today that is powerful to you.
What does it make you do or feel?

34. **SOMEONE ELSE'S PERSPECTIVE**

Choose a person close to you – someone you may be annoyed with, have frequent arguments with, or occasionally just don't get along with. Step into their shoes for just a moment. What does life look like from where they're standing? What's important and what isn't? Try to remember what this felt like the next time you meet.

35. **EVERYDAY MICRO-MINDFULNESS**

Choose a daily habit, such as brushing your teeth, drinking coffee, or taking the train, and – while doing it – simply pause and pay attention. Allow yourself to be fully in the moment. Try to make it a daily habit to be mindful in that same situation – you'll feel the difference in no time.

36. TWO-MINUTE WORKOUT: PLANK AWAY

Focus on either a knee-supported or push-up-style
plank and see how long you can hold your position.
If you're a beginner, try a thirty-second plank four times.
If you're more advanced, hold your plank for two
minutes straight. How long can you go? **Dani**

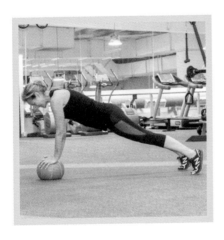

37. **START THE DAY RIGHT**

Breakfast is boss, so give it some love today. If you get this right, you'll be prepared for the day. The key to a winning breakfast is to try to mix it up and eat from as many of the food groups as possible so you get a good balance. And don't eat the same thing every day. The ideal breakfast is packed with a combination of whole grains, fruits, vegetables, dairy, and protein – a great example is a bowl of porridge made with milk, topped with fresh fruit, nuts, and seeds. **Jamie**

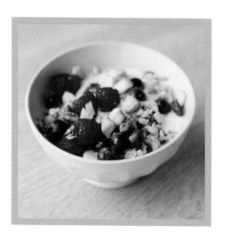

38. **NOTICE YOUR HUNGER**

Before eating, take a moment to notice what hunger feels like in your body. Remember how wonderful it is that you get to enjoy food in order to satisfy your body's needs. Next time you're hungry, pause and appreciate the feeling of anticipation for your meal. **Darya**

39. **TWO-MINUTE WORKOUT: WALL SIT**

For this easy workout you don't even need a chair – just a wall. Slowly slide your back down a wall until your thighs are parallel to the ground. Make sure your knees are directly above your ankles and keep your back straight. Work up to holding the position for two sets of sixty seconds. **Dani**

40. **DECLUTTER IN FIVE MINUTES**

Reducing clutter helps you gain clarity and paves the way for better routines. We all have lots of stuff we no longer need, but it can seem overwhelming to deal with a whole cabinet or box. So open a drawer and spend five minutes choosing just a handful of things to toss. **Caroline**

41. **BE GRATEFUL**

This micro-action can unlock vast reserves of well-being. We tend to think about life in relative terms – was today better than yesterday, am I doing better than my colleague, where am I in relation to my goals? Be grateful. Don't dwell on what you're lacking but be happy for what you have.

FOOD

42. TRY SOMETHING NEW

Get adventurous today and eat an ingredient you've
never tried before. Most of us buy the same stuff, week in,
week out, year in, year out. So it's time to mix things up.
Today, choose something – fruit, vegetable, cheese, fish,
meat, grain, or spice – you've never picked up before and
try it. Have fun! **Jamie**

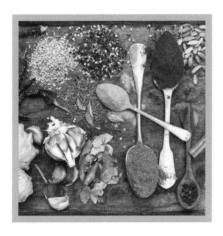

43. **CHOOSE WHOLE GRAINS**

Choose a whole grain option today. Eating whole grains regularly will make a massive difference to your health – they are powerful little things and can reduce the risk of strokes and heart disease. Without getting too geeky, they remain whole when they're processed, whereas refined grains lose lots of their nutrients during milling. Also, whole grains take longer to digest, which helps to keep us feeling fuller for longer. I also find that whole grain varieties such as whole wheat bread or brown rice give excellent texture and often have a deeper flavor, so they're great for adding an extra level to your meal. Double pleasure. **Jamie**

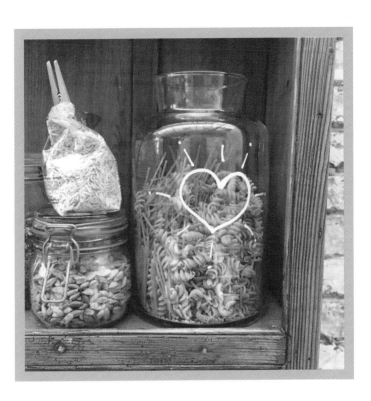

44. **ONE-MINUTE DIARY**

Take less than a minute to write down one thing that happened today. Keeping long diary entries every day is a resolution that a lot of us fail at, so make this short and manageable. What may seem like an ordinary or insignificant moment today can become a dear memory years from now.

....

....

....

....

....

....

....

....

FOOD

45. **EAT THE RAINBOW**

Have a colorful meal today (but keep it natural!).
A lot of info flies around about how to get all the vitamins
and minerals you need for optimal health, well-being, and
mood. But let's break it down: the simplest, easiest, most
effective way to ensure you're getting your fill of the good
stuff is to eat the rainbow. Different colored veggies and
fruits give us a whole range of different nutrients.
The more fresh, seasonal color on your plate,
the better – so mix it up! **Jamie**

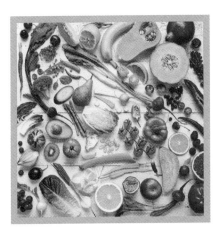

46. **EXPLORE THE NEIGHBORHOOD**

Put on your walking shoes and go out to explore your surroundings. Notice something new. Find a place you haven't visited before. Admire something for a second longer than usual. When you are paying attention to what's around you and get lost in the moment you may not only experience something new but also end up walking that extra mile.

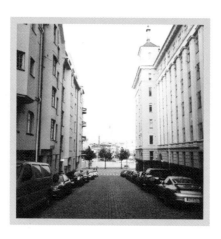

47. **TAKE QUALITY TIME**

Today, take some quality time. It may be time for yourself
doing something you love – read, write, work on a building
or gardening project. It may be for pampering yourself – take a
bath, enjoy the sun, put your feet up. Or it may be time spent
with your loved ones. Make it quality time and make it count.

48. **LIGHTEN YOUR PAPER LOAD**

Without noticing it, we tend to acquire a lot of unnecessary
things, which we then carry around. Go through your briefcase,
handbag, wallet, or pockets and get rid of old papers,
receipts, extra notebooks, and journals. Clearing your bag
is like clearing your mind. **Caroline**

49. **IMPROVE A HABIT**

Today is not about lofty resolutions but about improving an existing one. What habit are you trying to work on and how could you make it stick even better? Set yourself reminders, ask a friend for support, set smaller goals, or invest in those cool new sneakers to inspire your next workout. Whatever helps.

50. **SIT DOWN TWICE**

You may look a little odd but when sitting down today, even just at your desk or to watch TV, do it twice. We spend a lot of time sitting, which leaves our glutes underused. They are the largest muscles in our bodies, and going from sitting to standing activates our glutes, quads, and hamstrings. Double up: sit down twice! **Jamie S**

51. **ASSIGN A SURFACE A PURPOSE**

Surfaces are clutter magnets. We drop mail, bags, keys, and loose change anywhere handy. While you don't need to put everything away immediately, making sure that surfaces don't become catch-alls is important. Mail doesn't belong on a kitchen island; a comb and brush aren't useful on a desk. Today, rearrange what's on one surface in your life so that it serves a specific purpose. You'll be more organized in minutes. **Caroline**

52. **FORGIVE YOURSELF**

Regrets and self-reproach can weigh you down – they don't call it "emotional baggage" for nothing! Focus on an old regret or an old faux pas and give yourself a break – forget about it. What has passed has passed, but the future is right now. Make that future brighter – forgive yourself and move forward. **Caroline**

53. **A MEAL TO SHARE**

It's all about the love, baby! Share some food with a loved one. Whether it's a romantic proposition or quality time with a dear old friend, we all know that the way to someone's heart is often through their stomach. Make the time this week to cook a delicious meal from scratch that you can share. **Jamie**

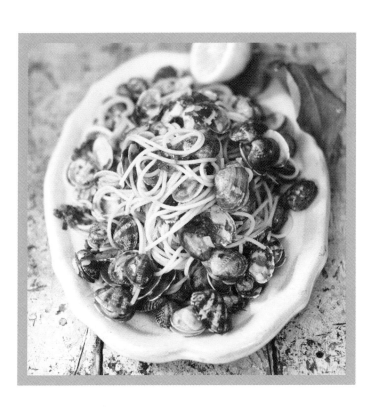

54. **TAKE IT ALL IN**

Take a moment to take it all in. When we're busy we often rush from one thing to the next and forget to stop and appreciate our surroundings. And that's really the easiest mindfulness exercise you can do. Take in the nature around you, appreciate your colleagues, observe your family from a distance, or admire the night sky. Whatever you do – be in the moment.

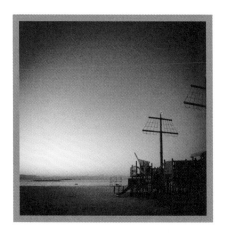

55. **SHAKE IT OFF**

A happy and healthy lifestyle starts with the right attitude.
What's an old attitude you're shaking off and what are
you replacing it with? Don't hurry through this one;
make it count for you.

Write it here:

....

....

....

....

....

....

....

....

56. **CHECK YOUR POSTURE**

Most of us spend a lot of the day sitting, which negatively impacts our posture. It means muscles aren't being used in the way they were designed. Correcting your posture can activate and strengthen muscles that have switched off. When you sit, sit at attention! Standing, pinch your shoulder blades together and pull down. Try sitting with good posture as long as possible without back support. Walk with your head held high. **Jamie S**

57. **READ FOR FIVE MINUTES**

Picking up a book for even a few minutes is a great habit. We love films, TV, and the world of content on our smartphones, but acknowledge that a good book is best for giving your mind both a rest and some stimulation. Pick up a book or magazine; relax and just read for a few minutes. How could you make reading for five minutes a day a new habit?

FOOD

58. STOP WHEN YOU'RE FULL

Today, stop eating when you're full (and I'm talking full, not stuffed!). It sounds simple but a lot of us eat until we've finished everything on our plate, as opposed to when we're no longer hungry. Maybe it's because we still have our parents' voices ringing in our ears telling us not to leave the table until our plates are clean! Try and combat that old message today, keeping any leftovers for another meal. **Jamie**

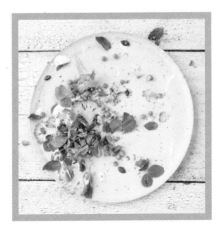

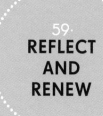

59·
**REFLECT
AND
RENEW**

For this Reflect and Renew micro-action,
think about what you have learned so far.

What has been most insightful?

Which micro-action has been your favorite?

Are you ready to change your Keep It Up action?

60. **LEFT OR RIGHT?**

We can get quite stuck in our ways, always typing on our tablets with the same hand, always holding our knife and fork in the same hand, etc. Doing something with your nondominant hand is great stimulus for your brain. So try it today: write a few sentences, eat a meal, or brush your teeth. You might even find it surprisingly fun! **Tara**

61. **SHOPPING BAG WEIGHT TRAINING**

Often it's really the small opportunities to move that are the best. When I go shopping with the kids, holding the bags becomes a bicep curl workout. Ditch the cart, hold your shopping bags, and do some bicep curls as you walk to the car. **Dani**

62. **STAND UP**

Standing is great for us and we should endeavor to minimize sitting time. So today, stand up. This is a great example of how micro becomes macro: standing for three extra hours a day, five days a week, for one year uses the same energy as running ten marathons! **Jamie S**

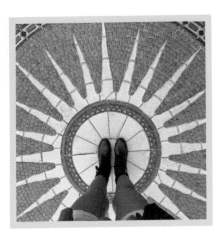

FOOD

63. **SIT AT THE TABLE**

We're a constantly distracted generation. How many of you are eating while reading this book? Or usually munch breakfast while checking emails, or grab lunch on the go, or have a few too many TV dinners? Food is one of life's simplest pleasures. You're much more likely to overeat if your mind is elsewhere. So sit at a table for your meals today. **Jamie**

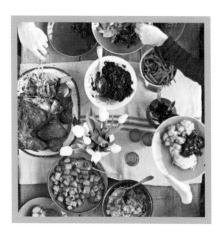

64. QUIET DOWN FOR FIVE MINUTES

Even if you enjoy being busy, taking a quiet moment once in a while is a really good habit to get into. Put everything aside and take a few minutes to refocus. Relax. Try to do nothing and enjoy it.

65. ACTIVATE YOUR ABS

If you don't use it, you lose it. While you are, for example, making breakfast or on the bus, pull your belly button in. This micro-action is amazing for your lower back as it activates the deep abdominal muscles that are usually asleep but help provide support. Activate your deep abs without effort today. **Jamie S**

FOOD

66. GET FRUITY

Keeping it super simple, just eat some fresh fruit today.
Too many of us don't, and those of us who do can easily get
stuck in a rut with what we choose. Fruit has loads of amazing
nutritional benefits, plus it's delicious and pretty much the
simplest snack there is. The more varied we keep our choices,
the more benefits we get – so mix it up and eat the rainbow.
Jamie

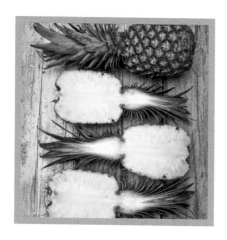

67. **THINK POSITIVE**

Almost everything we do starts as a thought, and
each thought impacts how we think, act, and feel.
Today, take control and consciously think more positively
about something. Positive thinking accumulates – people
who are primed to think positively see more possibilities,
take on activities, and develop skills a negative thinker
would not. If you want to learn more about the power of
positive thinking, there are some amazing talks on
the subject at ted.com.

68. **MAKE YOURSELF LAUGH**

Humor doesn't just boost your mood, it's good for the
body, too. Laughing stimulates your heart, lungs, and muscles,
and releases endorphins in your brain. So today, make sure you
enjoy a good laugh.

FOOD

69. **GUILTY HABITS**

Today, tackle one of those little guilty habits that can sometimes hold you back from positive change. We've all got them, whether it's going in for an extra helping or sneaking another cookie from the jar when you think no one's looking. Which of your guilty pleasures can you tackle today? Perhaps you're a breakfast-skipper or a kid's-dinner-finisher. Be bold and make a change. **Jamie**

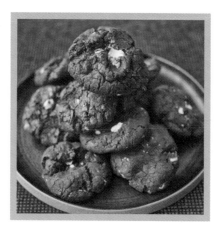

70. **REACH OUT TO SOMEONE**

We all have those friends or relatives we've wanted to call for a long time. How about seizing the moment and reaching out to them today? Grab the phone, write a message, pay them a visit, send them a gift, or just text a smiley face.

71. **LEAVE YOURSELF A NOTE**

Write a positive or uplifting note to yourself for tonight. Leave it on the fridge, the kitchen table, or ready to be found when you go to bed. If you can't think of anything to say to yourself, leave a note for someone else!

72. **MODIFY ONE MORNING HABIT**

Mornings can be a hassle. Take some time today to run through your current morning routine in your mind. What's working and what isn't? Find one thing you could improve in the mornings. For example, pick up the habit of reading the news, add in five minutes of meditation, prepare your clothes the night before, or simply leave home ten minutes earlier.

73. **TWO-MINUTE WORKOUT: WALL SQUATS**

Find a wall, face it, and stand approximately one foot away. Place your hands behind your head, bend down slowly, and do as many squats as you can in two minutes. How many can you do? **Dani**

74. **THE TWO-MINUTE RULE**

Quite simply, if something takes two minutes or less to complete, do it right away. Don't write it down, don't add it to your to-do list, just do it. It's surprising how many simple things we put off when we could get them done really quickly.

75. **BOOK BREAKFAST WITH A FRIEND**

When life gets busy with family, work, or studying, we often struggle to find enough time for friends. Mornings are a great time to meet as the day's tasks have yet to begin, so call up a friend and make a breakfast date.

76. DECIDE WHAT WON'T GET DONE TODAY

Many of us start each day with the assumption that we can get everything on our to-do list completed. As a result, we don't decide early enough what to put off and by the end of the day the choice has been made for us. Start today by deciding what won't get done, then focus like crazy on your short list. Part of mastering productivity is accepting the limits of your day and making conscious choices – before the day slips away.

Caroline

77. **TAKE A WALK**

Try taking short walks during the day to shake it up.
A two-minute walk in the office every twenty minutes can
be surprisingly beneficial to your health – research even shows
it can be more beneficial than an hour at the gym
after work! So get up, get out, and take a short walk.
For an added challenge, do not take your phone.

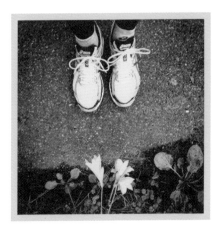

78. BEAUTIFUL FRESH HERBS

Today, use some fresh herbs in a dish. I've said before that if herbs didn't exist I'd probably give up cooking! They really are a complete joy and are key to taking any meal to the next level. Each one does its own incredible thing, and the more you experiment the more amazing combinations you'll discover. Woody herbs, such as rosemary, thyme, and sage, are excellent with meat and in the base of heartier dishes; and softer herbs, such as mint, basil, parsley, and coriander, are great in salads, in pastas, for sprinkling over dishes, or even for making your own pesto. **Jamie**

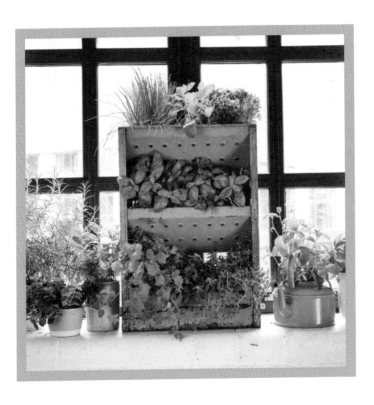

LOVE

79. WHAT DO YOU LIKE ABOUT YOURSELF?

We often spend so much time focusing on the small things
we're lacking or what we think is wrong that we forget
to see the good – especially when it comes to ourselves.
Take a moment and write down one thing you really like
about yourself. Whether it's a physical attribute, a skill
you have, or a strength – we all have something to be
proud of on a daily basis.

80. GET READY FOR BED EARLY

Get ready for bed well before bedtime. Wash your face, floss your teeth, soak your contacts, recharge your phone. Get it all done early so that as soon as you feel tired you can go straight to bed without having to do a single thing. **Caroline**

81. RETRO WALKING

Most commonly known as "backward walking," this originated in ancient China, where it was practiced for good health. When you walk backward, it puts less strain on your knee joints, making it ideal for people with knee problems or injuries. Also, because backward walking eliminates the typical heel strike to the ground (the toe contacts the ground first), it can lead to changes in pelvis alignment and help to open up the facet joints in your spine, potentially alleviating lower back pain in some people. So go backward! **Dani**

FOOD

82. EAT SEASONALLY

Eating bang-in-season fruit and vegetables means you get them at their best – they're super fresh, at their tastiest, and at their cheapest, too. Check out a calendar of seasonal foods, get inspired, and take your pick. Use one seasonal fruit or vegetable in a meal today. **Jamie**

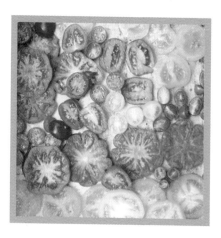

83. **FEEL AN EMOTION**

To create sustainable change you need to get engaged
emotionally as well as logically. The basic eight emotions
are fear, anger, disgust, shame, sadness, surprise, joy/
excitement, and love/trust. You can use these to get yourself
more or less engaged in an activity. Today, think how you
can use one of these feelings to your advantage. **Tara**

84. **SHARE SOMETHING THAT MAKES YOU LAUGH**

Found a funny picture on the internet? Or did you
hear a great joke? Share it with a friend today.
Sharing is caring and laughing is loving.

85. MAKE A SUSTAINABLE CHOICE

Make one green choice that shows the natural world some love. Here are a few ideas: opt out from paper junk mail or move to paperless billing. Get a reusable water bottle (50 billion water bottles are used annually, and only 20 percent get recycled). Reuse your plastic bags (1 trillion are used globally each year, and only 6 percent are recycled).

86. PREP ONE THING FOR TOMORROW

At any point during today, prepare one thing for tomorrow. Lay out your clothes, pack your backpack, prepare your lunch, or jump-start your breakfast. Whatever you prepare tonight will allow you to sleep a little longer and begin your day with less stress. Tomorrow morning is going to be a breeze. **Caroline**

87. **LOVE YOUR FREEZER**

Show your freezer some love. What I mean is, make the most of it! Your freezer is your best friend when it comes to saving waste and keeping healthy stuff in stock. One of my favorite things to do is chop up fruit that's just past its prime, bag it up in portions, and freeze it. Whiz it up as smoothies. Buying frozen vegetables is also great – they're often frozen really swiftly after being picked so nutrient-wise it's all still happening. Also you can just use what you need, when you need it. **Jamie**

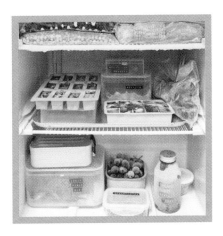

88.
REFLECT
AND
RENEW

Use this moment as motivation to renew your
commitments to yourself, particularly
your favorite micro-actions.

89. GO PAPERLESS FOR ONE NEW BILL

Have you been meaning to switch from paper bills to e-bills but
can never find the time? Today, select one monthly bill you
receive in the mail and opt for electronic billing instead. The
environment, your mailbox, and your sanity will thank you for it.
Caroline

90. FIND AN OLD PICTURE OF YOUR FAMILY

Do you have a box of photos from the days when pictures
were still taken on film, developed, and printed on paper?
Today, take a trip down memory lane and sort through
your old family photos. Pick your favorite and let
it remind you of days gone by.

91. **PLAN A WEEKEND ACTIVITY**

Make the most of an upcoming weekend by doing something
active. Plan something like going for a hike, for a walk, or
shopping on foot. Feeling frisky? Plan an adventure! No time?
Commit to ten push-ups on Saturday morning to get you going.
Jot down where you'd like to go here:

....

....

92. **CONCENTRATE ON LUNCH**

Take thirty minutes to enjoy your lunch away from your phone,
email, and other interruptions and you'll likely have a more
productive afternoon. The break will allow you to savor
your meal, consider afternoon priorities, and end your
day with greater vigor. **Caroline**

93. **COOK FROM SCRATCH**

If you cook from scratch and use lovely fresh ingredients,
you essentially have your health in your own hands. Cook a
meal from scratch today. Knowing how to cook is an essential
life skill. For any kitchen novices out there, having a few simple
recipes up your sleeve will serve you well for a lifetime, so get
your cookbooks out or get online and find a recipe that inspires
you to get in the kitchen. **Jamie**

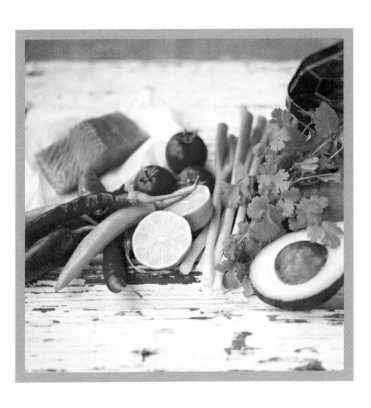

94. **THANK YOUR BODY**

Our bodies are incredibly intelligent and complex organisms that work hard to allow us to experience and enjoy life. Did you know that our hearts beat around 100,000 times a day? Yet it is easy to focus on the negative, especially if sickness shadows our lives. Thank your body for all it does: its sense of taste that helps you enjoy delicious food, legs that take you to beautiful places, a voice you can express your thoughts with, skin that keeps you protected, or muscles to carry groceries or hug a loved one. Cherish your body and you will instantly feel better.

95. **SLOW THE BEAT**

Play music with a slow beat during mealtimes. You'll naturally tend to eat with the rhythm, so slow down and eat more mindfully by playing soft music. **Darya**

96. **TAKE A STRETCHING BREAK**

Interrupt whatever you're doing and stretch. One minute
is enough. Stretch your arms, legs, back, and neck. Even a quick
movement is good for both body and mind. **Jamie S**

97. **READ SOMETHING NEW**

Teachers encourage children to read a lot to help instill
the "story structure" so they learn to think in sequence
while their brain still has a lot of plasticity. For adults,
reading something new can improve your creativity – so
if you love novels, maybe go for nonfiction or even poetry
today, or try to learn something new. **Tara**

FOOD

98. PRIDE OF PLACE

If you're surrounded by beautiful, tempting fresh options, you're more likely to put them in your mouth! Move the good stuff to pride of place today. In my house we always have a well-stocked fruit bowl close at hand, give a big bowl of salad pride of place on the dinner table, and have jugs of water in the fridge chilled and ready to pour. Get shuffling! **Jamie**

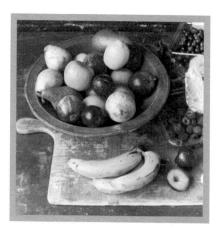

99. **LEARN A PLACE ON THE MAP**

Learning where places are not only improves your worldly wisdom but also keeps your brain active. Take a few minutes to study a map. Learn at least one new place. Can you pinpoint Ljubljana? The capital of Tibet? Kuopio?

100. **DROP SOME EMOTIONAL BAGGAGE**

Give up an old grudge, forgive a friend or colleague for something, stop dwelling on an old regret, or apologize to someone you've treated unfairly. Old emotional business weighs you down – they don't call it "baggage" for nothing. Today, target some old business and forgive, forget, and move forward. **Caroline**

101. **WORK AROUND THE HOUSE**

Do a few small tasks that take you around the house. We all have those little things we know we should fix, improve, start, or finalize – and ticking things off our to-do list can help get us moving, too. Is it a leaking faucet, a light bulb that needs changing, a plant that needs watering, or that pile of leaves in the garden you could gather up? Put on your work boots and complete a few small tasks that get you moving.

102. **IMPROVE YOUR SLEEP ENVIRONMENT**

Sleep is when your brain rests. It's when your muscles relax and develop. It's also when you replenish your energy stores to take on the world again the next day. What small improvement could you make to your sleep environment to ensure a better night's sleep?

103. **YOUR POSITIVE MANTRA**

We spend much of our time fretting about the negatives instead of focusing on the positives. Get in front of the mirror today and tell your reflection a positive mantra. For example: "Happiness isn't size-specific," "Work out because you love your body, not because you hate it," or "I am strong, I am beautiful, I am enough." What are you telling yourself today?

104. **CLEAN UP ONE THING**

Wipe down the fridge, straighten a corner of your desk, clean the keyboard on your laptop, or return stray items to the medicine cabinet. It's amazing how five minutes of cleanup can change your entire outlook and make life feel manageable again. **Caroline**

105. **A CHILDHOOD FOOD HABIT**

The earlier we learn good food habits the better – good habits learned young make for a healthier, happier life. Think back and identify one of the good food habits you picked up as a child. Was it a meal you learned to cook that you still make today? Perhaps you were nagged about eating your greens and it's stuck? Whatever it is, celebrate that positive habit and keep it up! **Jamie**

....

....

....

....

....

....

....

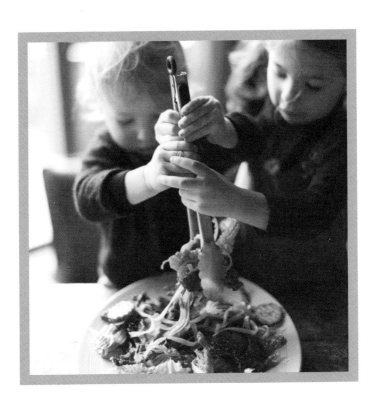

106. **GO NUTS**

Today, pay homage to the wonderful world of nuts. They're incredible – deliciously diverse in flavor, packed with beneficial unsaturated fats and lots of essential vitamins and minerals, and will give you an energy boost. Try just a small handful as a snack or added to a meal – pecans on oatmeal, pine nuts over pasta, or crushed walnuts over a salad. And if nuts won't do, a sprinkle of seeds is also a really good way to go. **Jamie**

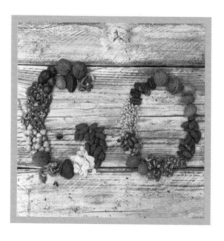

107. DELEGATE ONE THING

One key to greater productivity is delegation. Most of us take on too much and only think of delegating when it's too late. Today, identify one item you can delegate. It might be a duty for an upcoming social event, asking someone at work to write up the key points of a meeting, or getting your child to set the table. Delegating is a skill. It takes practice to learn how to spot a delegable item and get it on to someone else's to-do list before it's too late. **Caroline**

108. GO TO SLEEP FIFTEEN MINUTES EARLIER

There is no greater productivity boost than sleep. Sleep restores the key mental resources of willpower, decision-making, and active initiative. Sleep rebalances hormones for steady energy. Sleep allows your subconscious to make new connections and discoveries that will support your problem-solving. Even just fifteen minutes more sleep can make a big difference. **Caroline**

109. **WALK AN EXTRA MILE**

One mile is approximately 1.6 kilometers and about 2,000 steps. Could you get off the bus a stop or two earlier, park the car further away, add in an after-lunch walk, take your phone calls while pacing around, or resolve to always walk up the stairs? Try to achieve it one or more days this week. Small changes really do add up over time. **Jamie S**

110. **FIND KINDNESS AROUND YOU**

The science behind how witnessing happiness can affect our well-being is fascinating. Today, stop, look around, and notice small acts of kindness. Is it a person, item, service, or moment? Where can you find kindness today? Can't find it? Create it.

111. **FRUIT SWITCH**

I can't go on enough about fruit – it's nature's genius way of making it easy to get the good stuff into your diet. Today, switch up your usual fruit choice. Whether you have a banana at breakfast, grab an apple at 11 AM, or blitz up the same smoothie combo each morning, challenge yourself today to choose a fruit you don't usually pick. Each fruit has a different nutritional makeup, so do your body a favor and mix things up – it's also a treat for the taste buds. Choose something seasonal so it's at its tastiest and best! **Jamie**

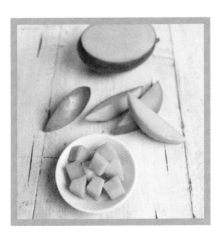

112. **PARK BENCH OR CHAIR STEP-UP**

Find opportunities outside or at home to do small bursts of movement. Here's a simple one: when you are out and about and spot a bench, or in your home with a chair, do step-ups. Step up with one foot, then the other, and repeat fifteen times on each foot. This will tone your legs and get your heart pumping. **Dani**

113. **EAT WITH GRATITUDE**

Take a few seconds before you eat to remember all the people and resources that went into creating your meal. Appreciate the farmers, the soil, the sunshine, the water, the shops, and, yes, yourself as well. **Darya**

114. **MAKE SOMEONE ELSE SMILE**

Spread the joy by making someone else smile. Everyone feels
lonely at times, so try to think of someone who might need some
cheering up – be that a loved one or a complete stranger.
The reward center of the brain actually gets a stronger
dopamine hit when we make someone else smile first.

115. **READ ONE PIECE OF NEWS**

Do you know what's happening in the world? In your home
country or town? Open a news site, skim through, and read
at least one full article. Reading the news helps you gain
perspective and can take your mind off your own challenges.

116.
REFLECT
AND
RENEW

In this review, write down three things you want to be remembered for.

Reflecting on what you want to be remembered for can increase your level of happiness and give you perspective on life.

Does your vision fit with the person you are today?

FOOD

117. **GET CREATIVE WITH VEGGIES**

We all have a repertoire of dishes we whip up, week in, week out, but mixing things up and getting inspired with new recipe ideas are crucial to keeping veggies on your menu long term. Today, get creative with vegetables. Switch up salads by using a speed peeler to add ribbons of zucchini and carrots, or grate a load of gorgeous fresh veggies to make a slaw. Use your imagination and have fun! **Jamie**

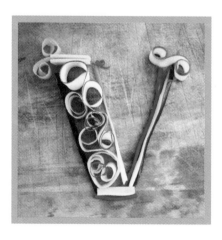

118. **VOLUNTEER FOR SOMETHING**

Volunteering is a great way to help those in need around you. You'll feel great, too, for doing something that really matters. So help out a friend, volunteer to carry your neighbor's shopping up the stairs, or do some research into volunteer opportunities close by.

119. **TWO-MINUTE WORKOUT: EVENING STRETCH**

Take two minutes to truly stand silent and listen to your breathing, then start with some light stretches to get your muscles moving and your blood flowing. Our seated or standing positions throughout the day can tense up our muscles, and those tensions need to be released. **Dani**

120. **BE A TOURIST IN YOUR HOMETOWN**

Traveling expands our thinking and gives us perspective.
But why not get the same effect without leaving your own town?
There are a lot of new things to experience and see if you look
through the eyes of a tourist. Go out today and explore.

121. **TAKE A WALK AT LUNCH**

Walking for just eight minutes can improve creativity
and problem-solving for hours afterwards. A brisk walk
after lunch will also boost your metabolism and prevent
that midafternoon slump that can hit us both in the
workplace and at home. **Caroline**

122. **CREATE A DREAM PAGE**

Dream boards are a great way to visualize your aspirations. Fill this page, or use the space below, with writing and doodles to make them concrete. This is a great escape when you need it, and making things visual may just give you that extra little nudge you need to pursue what you wish for.

123. **KEEP YOUR WATER BOTTLE OR GLASS FILLED**

Water boosts brain function and physical stamina, and helps keep ideas and energy flowing all day. The trick to drinking more is simply to always have water within reach. Practice keeping your glass filled all day today. **Caroline**

124. **MEASURE MINDFULLY**

We have lots of ways to measure ourselves. Many people weigh themselves, count their calories consumed, hours slept, steps walked, etc. – but it can become obsessive. So cut back on counting and measure only one or a few things that really matter. Or just listen to your body. Be mindful of how you feel and whether you need a rest. **Jamie S**

125. NOTICE AN ANIMAL, TREE, OR FLOWER

Nature is amazing, but we rarely notice just how amazing.
Watch a documentary or, even better, go outside and
explore nature. Find a flower, a tree, or an animal
and look up its name.

126. LEARN ONE THING ABOUT HOW YOUR BODY WORKS

Knowing how the body works is key to making it work better
for you. So open a dictionary or a book or browse some reliable
websites and learn about the human body. What interesting
fact can you find that helps you treat your body better?

FOOD

127. GET-AHEAD GRUB

Today, prepare one thing to save you time and stress over the next few days. You could try cooking a big batch of super-healthy grains to toss through lunch-box salads, or freeze portions of fruit ready to blitz into an easy breakfast smoothie. I love to get a big pot on the stove and make a hearty ragu to toss through pasta, have on toast, or freeze for a lasagna. What can you do to make meals a little bit easier this week? **Jamie**

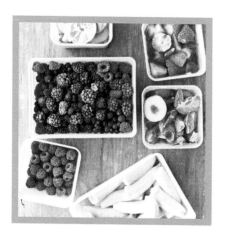

128. **COMPLIMENT A STRANGER**

Have you ever had a stranger on the street compliment your
outfit or your looks? Did you get an endorphin rush that lasted
for the rest of the day? Make it your mission to compliment
a stranger today. It may be a complete stranger on the bus
for something they're wearing, the barista at your favorite café
for his or her coffee-making skills, or that stylish older
gentleman living next door to you. There's a guaranteed
good feeling for you, too.

129. **LISTEN TO CLASSICAL MUSIC**

Classical music has been shown to reduce blood pressure,
reduce stress and anxiety, and improve sleep quality. Put on
some classical tunes and unwind. What are you listening to?

LOVE

130. **SUBJECT MATTERS**

We all have at least one topic we're knowledgeable about.
Be it history, Japanese gardening, mathematical theories,
World War II, or parenting techniques – it's your game.
What is your favorite subject? Today, consider how you
can better cultivate that knowledge in your daily life.

MOVE

131. **MOVE TOGETHER**

Moving together keeps you more accountable and makes
it more fun. Team up with a friend for a light jog in the park,
schedule a joint workout with your significant other, or join
a group class. If you have kids, make your joint time active – go
walking, skating, surfing, cycling, or visit the park. **Dani**

132. **ENJOY A SMALL ACHIEVEMENT**

Research has shown that it's small, frequent boosts of joy
that lead to happiness, not the rare big stuff. It's the little
things in daily life that have the power to make lasting
improvements to our happiness. So celebrate a small
achievement today – having your favorite lunch, moving
for just five minutes, choosing a book instead of your
iPad, or receiving a smile from someone you like.

133. **SAY "THANK YOU"**

Say "thank you" to someone today. Two such simple
words that we often forget. Do you remember an occasion
where someone thanked you and how good that felt?
Thank someone – a friend, a colleague, a family member,
or even someone working at your local supermarket.

FOOD

134. SNACK SMART

Today's micro-action is to eat a tasty, healthy snack that will spank your taste buds and subdue hunger. People often ask me if snacking is good or bad – well, let me clarify that snacking is absolutely good. It helps keep your blood sugar levels in check, which means you stay alert and active. But it's got to be the good stuff – I'm talking fruit, nuts, seeds, a little salad, something nice and nutritious rather than diving into the cookie jar. **Jamie**

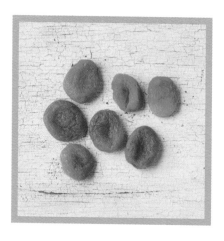

135. **SHOW LOCAL SOME LOVE**

Get out in your local area and appreciate your surroundings.
Find a street you haven't walked down before, poke
around some independent shops, or admire the buildings
around you. Try to look at your neighborhood as if
seeing it for the first time.

136. **ALLOW TIME FOR BOREDOM**

In a world of constant stimulation, we flip channels incessantly,
immediately pick up our phone when we're alone, or always
have the TV or radio on in the background. But boredom can
be a stimulus for change. In fact, studies show that boredom
boosts creativity as it motivates us to approach new and
rewarding activities. So today – give boredom a chance!

FOOD

137. FIFTY SHADES OF GREEN

Go one step further with "eating green" today and make half of one meal green veggies. The more varied you make your greenage the better, and it doesn't have to be a chore – you can sneak greens into all sorts of dishes. Think adding a handful of peas to rice, stirring spinach into mash, or adding a dollop of homemade guacamole to a meal. Upping your greens will help keep your body ticking. (Even green chiles are packed with vitamin C, which is music to my ears!) **Jamie**

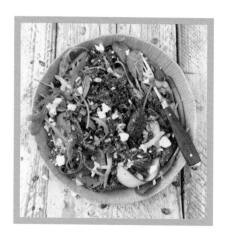

138. **WHAT DID YOU ACCOMPLISH TODAY?**

Take a moment and look back on today. What did you accomplish? Write down something that felt good and why.

....

....

....

....

....

....

....

....

....

139. **SIT WITH YOUR TEA OR COFFEE**

Make your drink of choice, then sit down for a few minutes.
No phone, no paper, just sit and think about your week. Source
physical energy from your drink and mental
energy from a moment of stillness.

140. **TWO-MINUTE WORKOUT: PELVIC FLOOR**

Pelvic-floor muscle exercises are important for both men
and women, and are very useful to prevent incontinence,
particularly for women who have had children. Sit, stand,
or lie down with your legs slightly apart and relax your thighs,
buttocks, and abdomen muscles. Tighten the muscles around
your front and back passages, drawing the pelvic-floor muscles
up inside. Develop this into a daily habit by doing it while you
are stirring your dinner, brushing your teeth, or about to go
to bed. Consistency is key. **Dani**

141. **PREP ONE THING**

"Failing to plan is planning to fail" – so the saying goes.
At some point today, prep something for a meal for tomorrow.
It doesn't matter whether it's marinating some meat or fish
overnight, making an extra portion of your supper for
tomorrow's lunch, or soaking some oats for an overnight
oatmeal in the morning. A little bit of planning can save you
time, stress, and money – enjoy. **Jamie**

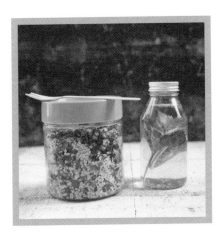

142. **GET VITAMIN D – GO OUTSIDE!**

Sunshine – how we love it. It's the best source of vitamin D,
which is produced when sunlight hits the skin. So get outside
to fuel up – and why not take a brisk walk while you're at it!

143. **SET A TECH RULE**

Technology brings us many wonderful things, but it can be
a distraction from real life, and deep down many of us know
we're a bit addicted. So today, set a clear tech-timeout rule.
No phones or TV at the dinner table? No digital devices after
9 PM? Only checking email once per hour? Turning off all alerts
when you leave the office? Write down your chosen rule here:

....

....

144. **ENJOY A MEAL**

Walking or driving while eating can make it feel like you aren't having a meal at all. And research confirms that you're more likely to overeat when you're distracted by another task. Take the time to sit down and really savor your food today. You deserve it. **Darya**

145. **SET A GO-TO-SLEEP ALARM**

We use alarm clocks to get us up in the morning, but for many the challenge is actually the night before – going to bed early enough. So try this. Decide on a bedtime (count seven to eight hours back from your wake-up time) and set an alarm for when it's time to go to sleep.

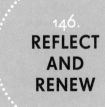

146.
REFLECT
AND
RENEW

Today, reflect on what type of micro-actions work best for you.

Recall an instance when you've really felt that a micro-action has positively impacted your day and consider why that was.

Have you repeated that micro-action yet?

If not, today's the day to do so!

147. BALANCED BREAKFAST

I'm sure we've all heard over and over that breakfast is the most important meal of the day, and let me tell you, it really is! Show breakfast the love it deserves and eat a balanced meal today. Make it a joy, not a chore – try pimping your oatmeal with a sprinkle of cinnamon, whizzing up a beautiful berry smoothie, or cracking out some eggs. Whatever you do, enjoy it! **Jamie**

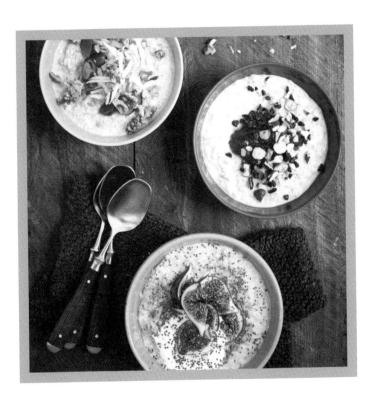

148. **A STRENGTH OF YOURS**

What's one thing you're really good at? Take a moment of reflection and write it down. It may be your ability to think positively, your "can do" attitude, effective working practices, a magically intuitive empathy, or your brilliant analytical skills. Whatever your strengths are, identifying them makes you more likely to actively use them and strengthen them even further!

....

....

149. **ONE ROOM DECOR**

Decorating your home is rewarding work but may feel like a huge chore. Pick one room in your home (or just one part of one room) and address that. Shift around the placement of furniture, add a fun new item, play around with different colors, or simply rearrange a bookshelf to look nice.

150. **USE UP ONE THING**

Around the world, we throw out 1.3 billion tons of edible food every year. That seems crazy to me, so today get food smart and do your bit to help reduce that massive figure. Use up one food item that was destined for the trash. If you've got bread that's seen softer days, tear it up and bake it to make croutons or blitz it into bread crumbs for sprinkling on a pasta dish. Create a lovely jumbled-up chopped salad from odds and ends in your vegetable drawer or simply chuck some fruit in the freezer ready to stew up for an easy dessert. **Jamie**

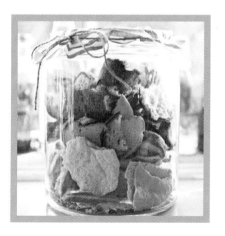

151. **HEALTHY HEART**

To keep our hearts nice and healthy, it's important to keep our intake of saturated fat below 20 g a day. Do one thing today to reduce your saturated-fat intake. I often swap the butter on my toast for avocado (I love butter, but everything in moderation).

What can you do? Here are a few tips: measure oil with a measuring spoon to give you more control over the amount you use, trim away the excess fat from meat, or skim away any fat that rises to the top of meaty stews. You can also grill, poach, boil, steam or bake food – and, my favorite, use yogurt instead of cream wherever possible. **Jamie**

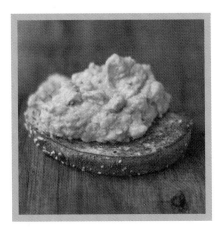

152. ENJOY AN INSPIRATION

Get inspired. Trigger new thoughts. Let your mind wander.
Think outside the box. What inspires you? Music? Art?
A teacher? A book? Your mother's words of wisdom?
Choose an inspiration and enjoy it.

153. PRETEND IT'S THE WEEKEND

What do you love the most about weekends? The stress-free
Friday mode? Making banana pancakes in the morning?
Eating a delicious Saturday night dinner? Reading books
during the day? Meeting with friends and family? We naturally
have more time on the weekend, but there are many small
things we can do during the week to enjoy life a bit more. So,
today, add one weekend feature into your day!

154. **TELL SOMEONE YOU LOVE THEM**

Putting our feelings into words and expressing them
to our loved ones is something many of us struggle with.
But don't take love for granted – reminding the loved
ones in your life (and yourself) that you love them by
saying so not only makes you and them feel good,
but will also strengthen the bond between you. Today,
tell someone in your life that you love them.

155. **STOCK UP ON ONE SUPPLY**

Zero in on a staple supply that you often run out of at
the last minute and stock up on it now. Toilet paper, cat food,
printer paper, ink, or light bulbs. Either stop by the store or
go online – get a little bit ahead on supplies and watch
your stress level decline. **Caroline**

156. **FRIDAY PREP FOR NEXT WEEK**

What's one thing you can do on Friday that's going
to make Monday easier? Fill the car up with gas? Iron
an outfit ready for work? Get a load of laundry done?
Stock up on lunch items? Think of one thing that trips you
up on Monday morning and prepare for it this Friday. You'll
enjoy the weekend more and you'll have more energy next
week if you take care of it in advance. **Caroline**

157. **WEAR WHAT MAKES YOU FEEL GOOD**

What you wear can have a really big impact on your
mood, self-image, and confidence. Put a little extra effort
into what you wear today and choose clothes that make
you feel really good. Be it that new dress, a smart suit, warm
woolen socks, or your favorite old T-shirt.

158. **TWO-MINUTE WORKOUT: BURPEES**

Burpees are one of the most effective full-body exercises around. Try and bust out as many burpees as you can to lift your heart rate. This is an excellent two-minute morning workout to get the day started. Don't know what a burpee is? Look up a tutorial video online. **Dani**

159. **SKIP A COMPLAINT**

At some point today, you may be tempted to complain – about the weather, travel, a family member, or office politics. Instead of giving in to sounding off, see what it does for your mind and spirit to just let the moment pass without comment.

160. **TAKE A "THINKING TEN"**

Tackling your to-do list day after day puts the brain in "execution" mode. That's great, but make sure you are doing the right things. Take a "thinking ten" today and reflect on your priorities for ten minutes.

....

....

....

....

....

....

....

....

161. **IT'S A WRAP**

One thing we can all do to minimize waste generated by food
is to cut down on packaging. Don't worry if you aren't a great
composter or your kitchen is stuffed with shopping bags. Today,
just remember to recycle or, even better, reuse one piece
of food packaging. Keep a hummus container to pack snacks
for on the go, use plastic bags as trash can liners, or, if you
want to go really green, use an empty tin as a pot to grow fresh
herbs on your windowsill! **Jamie**

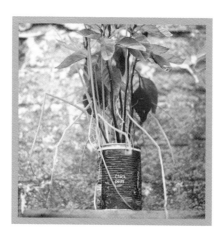

162. **REMEMBER A WOMAN IN YOUR LIFE**

Think of a woman who has had a big impact on you –
it can be someone who has been important at some point
in your life, or someone that you see every day – and extend
your appreciation to them. Call, send a message, or write
a letter to them; it will surely make their day.

163. **CHECK YOUR PHONE ONLY EVERY HALF HOUR**

The fight for mental real estate is fierce. We're constantly
assaulted by beeps, pop-ups, vibrations, and advertisements.
When we get into a meeting, we check our phone. When
we're cooking dinner, we stop to check our phone. We can't
control the environment, but we can control ourselves. Limit
yourself to phone checks only every half hour and see
what it does for your productivity. **Caroline**

164. **ONE EASY SWAP**

Today, swap one piece of food or drink for a healthier choice. We've all been there, made a vow to drastically change our eating habits and found ourselves face-first in the fridge at 10 PM. So instead of giving something up, just swap it out for a more nutritious option. The more realistic your habit changes are, the better chance they'll stick. **Jamie**

165. **TAKE A CAT NAP**

A five- to ten-minute nap in the afternoon works wonders on productivity for the rest of the day. The trick is finding a quiet and cozy place to take that nap. If you're at home, it's easy; at work, perhaps a little tricky. But with practice, you can learn to sleep almost anywhere. Set the timer on your phone and close your eyes. Even if you don't fall fully asleep, when you open your eyes you'll be refreshed. **Caroline**

FOOD

166. **SHOW-STOPPING SPICES**

Cooking from scratch with spices will elevate your cooking to the next level and help make it sing. Experiment with some new spices today. The right combo can turn a simple dish into something really special. They're also a really smart way to lower your salt intake as they are so packed with flavor, you can often get away with using less seasoning. **Jamie**

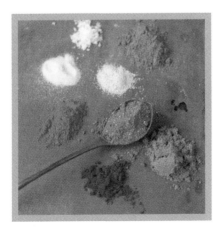

167. **SURGERY-FREE EYEBROW LIFTS**

Moving your face is like moving your body – it relaxes and tones muscles. For two minutes, lift your brows up and down (and try not to laugh too much). This exercise lifts and improves the shape of the brows: it reduces frown ridges and lines in between, opens up the eye area, and lifts the upper eyelid, reducing hooded and wrinkled eyes. The increased tone in the muscles over the scalp gives a general lifted effect to the forehead! **Dani**

168. **HELP OUT IN YOUR COMMUNITY**

To make a difference in the world we often think about global causes and lofty goals, but there are lots of opportunities to do this much closer to home. Find a cause in your own community where you can help out. Be it planting some flowers in a community garden, volunteering for a nonprofit organization, or helping your neighbor. Every act of kindness counts.

169. **WHAT'S BEST RIGHT NOW?**

On any given day, no matter what else might happen, there's always something positive to appreciate. It may be a situation, a feeling, something you did well, a kind word, or an event you're looking forward to. What's best right now for you?

Write it down here:

....

....

....

....

....

....

....

....

170. **QUICK KITCHEN CLEAR-UP**

Today, declutter one kitchen surface or cabinet. It doesn't have to be a proper deep clean, and no elbow grease will be needed. Just pick one area of your kitchen that hoards the most clutter and be brutal. Take no prisoners – banish anything that has nothing to do with cooking. (I'm looking at you, piggy banks and magazine racks!) Having your kitchen utensils close at hand and not surrounded by clutter will help you to be more instinctive and efficient in the kitchen. **Jamie**

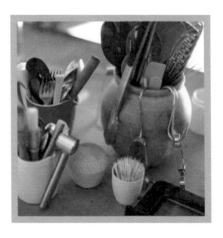

171. **TWO-MINUTE WORKOUT: HEEL KICKS**

To elevate your heart rate or bust a cardio workout, kick your heels up to your bottom and go hard for thirty seconds, then rest for ten seconds. Do this three times for a quick cardio session. **Dani**

172. **A CULTURAL EXPERIENCE**

Book tickets to the theater, make a plan to visit a museum, admire architecture, or pick up a classic book. This is soup for the soul. Cultural activities have been linked to increased well-being, so get out there and get cultural!

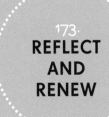

173·
REFLECT
AND
RENEW

Take a moment to celebrate the things that you've accomplished while working through this book.

Be honestly proud of how far you have come!

Then look ahead – what do you want to achieve before the end of the book?

Try to break that goal down into small micro-actions for the next phase.

174. **TEN-MINUTE "FUTURE DREAMING"**

For ten minutes, sit down in a quiet place and do some "future dreaming." No need to make any grandiose plans, just let your thoughts drift to a nice vision of the future. Where will you be? With whom? Doing what? What could you do today to get you closer to that vision?

Write some ideas down here:

FOOD

175. **SNACK ON A VEGGIE**

Keep it simple and snack on a veggie. Vegetables are
the unsung heroes of the snack world – they feature heavily
at lunch and dinner but are often kept on the snack sidelines.
It's pretty easy for bad snacking habits to slip under the
radar – even the most saintly of eaters can fall victim to that
4 PM sugar-fix snack attack. So today, when you need a
pick-me-up between meals, reach for a veggie. **Jamie**

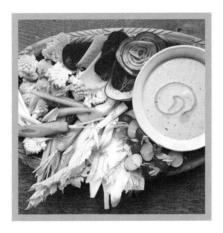

176. **TIDY UP**

Keeping order can be as simple as straightening things up
a little bit, often. Today, try to do this every time you leave a
room – whether it's the kitchen, the garage, or your desk/office
at work – tidy something up. Put a stray book back on the shelf,
smooth out a pile of papers, sweep coins off a dresser and into
your wallet. You'll be surprised at the difference it makes
to your surroundings and your mood. **Caroline**

177. **TWO-MINUTE WORKOUT: COUCH DIPS**

When a commercial comes on while watching TV, take
advantage of the pause to do sets of dips on the couch
or a chair. This is a great tricep workout that will help
to tone your arms where they wobble. **Dani**

178. **A MEMORY-FILLED SONG**

Music has amazing powers. It can stimulate old memories as vividly as if they happened yesterday. Take a trip down memory lane and listen to a song that reminds you of a person, situation, or beloved place.

179. **CLOUD GAZING**

Have you ever looked up at the sky and just stopped? Stopped because the clouds are displaying mesmerizing formations, the approaching rain clouds are strikingly dramatic, or you recognize a familiar shape in the clouds? Today – look up at the sky and do some cloud gazing. What do you see? Interesting shapes, colors, movement, the promise of better or worse weather? Allow yourself to get lost contemplating the sky.

180. **EVERYONE LOVES A MISFIT**

Most supermarkets reject fruit and vegetables that aren't perfect – 30 percent is wasted in the US alone. Today is all about embracing unusual fruit and vegetables to support our farmers. The natural stuff comes in all different shapes and sizes and is just as delicious and nutritious – no matter how it looks. Get creative and show your support to save waste.

181. **ORGANIZE THE MEDICINE CABINET**

Open your bathroom cabinet, pick one shelf, remove things that don't belong, wipe down the shelf and reorganize the remaining items – all in five minutes. Organizing just one shelf is fast, easy, and immediately reduces clutter. **Caroline**

182. **COZY UP AT HOME**

Today, curl up in a blanket with a book, have a mug of hot chocolate, lounge around on colorful pillows, or watch your favorite film to cheer you up! What is "cozy" to you?

183. **CONQUER A CRAVING**

Focus in on a craving for eating something unhealthy and satisfy it with a more wholesome choice. Life would be boring if we didn't indulge in tasty treats every now and again, but cravings can often get the better of us. For instance, instead of midafternoon chocolate, freeze some grapes to snack on, or swap that one-coffee-too-many for a therapeutic herbal tea. **Jamie**

FOOD

184. COOK DON'T CHUCK

Save an ingredient that's past its prime from being thrown away and use it in a meal. Got a few carrots nudging toward softness? Make a soup. There's a really geeky satisfaction that comes with using up food that would've otherwise been thrown out, and you're helping the planet, too. **Jamie**

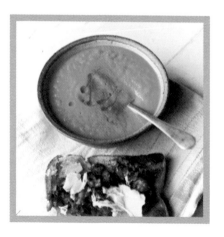

185. **SEEK OUT FEEDBACK**

Today, ask a colleague, family member, or friend for feedback.
Seeking out feedback at work inspires thoughtful responses
and boosts your standing by demonstrating that you are
dedicated to performing to the best of your ability. Asking
a friend, partner, or family member how you might improve
your approach to something creates trust and can give
you new personal insight. To improve, you don't have
to agree, just listen. **Caroline**

You might find it helpful to record the feedback here:

....

....

....

....

....

....

....

186. **PLAY WITH A BALL**

For today's workout, find your inner child and do something
involving a ball. Play tennis, juggle, play fetch with a dog,
challenge someone to a football game, or just play catch
against the wall by yourself. Enjoy! **Jamie S**

187. **A PHRASE IN A FOREIGN LANGUAGE**

Learning new languages is one of the best ways to increase
your brain's neuroplasticity as an adult. Today, flex the
language centers of your brain and learn a useful phrase
in another language. If there is a place you've always wanted
to go, learn to say "thank you" in that country's language.

188. ENJOY THE MOMENT

We tend to rush through routines, chores, and to-dos, always focusing on the next thing on our agenda. This can be good for getting things done, but we run the risk of forgetting to enjoy the moment. So today, pause and be present in what you're doing. It could be taking time over your morning coffee or tea, finding something funny, or relaxing with your feet up in the evening. What moment will you fully enjoy today?

....

....

....

....

....

....

189. **ENJOY A VIEW**

Today, simply enjoy a view. Taking in your surroundings is a great way to calm down, practice mindfulness, and enjoy a few minutes for yourself. What's a view you could enjoy today? A beach full of people? The view from your kitchen window? A busy street on your way to work? A familiar view in your city, or the view from the window of the bus? What do you see?

....

....

190. **A SONG YOU DANCE TO**

Today, play a song that makes you dance. You may be someone who can break out into dance at any appropriate (or inappropriate) moment, someone who dances alone while vacuuming, or a dedicated party dancer. Whoever you are, there's always that song that will get you grooving – so put it on and get down!

191. **PUT YOUR TO-DO LIST LAST**

End your day today by making tomorrow's to-do list.
This will help you put what you need to get done into
perspective and provide a visual reminder of your
priorities first thing in the morning. **Caroline**

Write tomorrow's to-do list here:

FOOD

192. MAKE A MEAT-FREE MEAL

We humans eat a lot of meat, and it's a huge drain on the environment. It takes more than 2,000 gallons of water to produce just two beef steaks, compared to under 35 gallons to produce 1 pound of potatoes – that's a big difference! Today, enjoy a meat-free meal. As well as being good for the environment, celebrating veggies will probably save you a bit of cash, too. **Jamie**

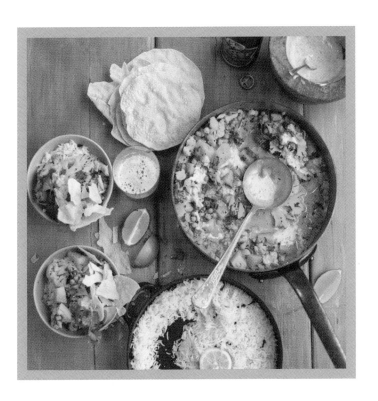

193. **COMPLIMENT YOURSELF**

Every thought and emotion creates a neurochemical reaction
that affects your well-being. Today, say a few words of
affirmation to yourself. What have you achieved recently
that you're proud of? What do you like when you look in
the mirror? Complimenting yourself gives you confidence,
balance, and a positive spin to the day.

194. **WHAT CALMS YOU DOWN?**

We all have our own ways of managing stress, of relaxing
and refocusing. What calms you down? Becoming aware of
the most effective way for you to calm down is an important first
step to start doing it more consciously and regularly.

195. **MAKE YOUR BED**

The simple act of making your bed in the morning can combat
the blues. This may sound strange, but it starts the day off on
the right track, gives a visual lift to the room, and makes it more
inviting to go to bed in the evening when the sheets aren't all
crumpled up from the night before. Try to make it a habit to
make your bed – it only takes two minutes.

196. **ENJOY SILENCE**

Take a moment and enjoy the silence. If you live in a city, you're probably surrounded by noise most of the time, but even outside the city we tend to fill up silences with different sounds such as TV, music, or radio. Make a conscious effort to find a silent place and enjoy the lack of sound. Give your mind the space to run free and fill the void itself.

197. **FAVORITE FRUIT**

Today is about celebrating gorgeous, seasonal, tasty, fresh fruit! Simply eat your favorite fruit. They all contain different vitamins, minerals, and nutrients, which help keep our bodies healthy, so a good philosophy to remember going forward is to mix up your choices! **Jamie**

198. ASK SOMEONE FOR ADVICE

Nothing builds a bridge like asking someone for their opinion or counsel, and getting someone else's perspective can help you make better decisions. Today, think about something you've been trying to solve by yourself and seek out someone's advice. Thinking of refinancing but don't know how to compare options? Wondering if you should seek flexible hours at work? Reaching out to a personal or professional connection for a conversation will not only help you solve a problem, but it will also strengthen a relationship that could prove invaluable.

What advice did you receive?

....

....

....

....

....

....

FOOD

199. **POWER UP WITH PLANT PROTEIN**

Meat and dairy are excellent sources of protein, but let's
not underestimate the power in plants! Today, eat some
protein-rich nuts, seeds, or grains, such as quinoa. Some
legumes are great plant-protein sources, too – think lovely
beans, lentils, and chickpeas. Protein is mega important – we
need it for growth, muscle repair, and brain function. **Jamie**

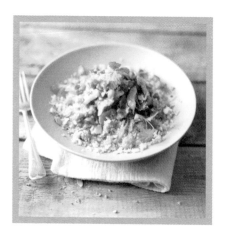

200. **A DISTANT MEMORY**

Take a moment to recall a distant memory. Your memory is a powerful tool — by sitting down and recollecting, you can resurrect strong emotions and thoughts. Recalling good memories vividly helps boost your overall happiness. So take a trip down memory lane to a positive event in your past.

201. **DO SOMETHING SILLY**

We can easily get into the macro-habit of taking life way too seriously. Small acts of silliness are the best cure — today, do something genuinely silly. Jump into a big puddle of water, climb a tree, play a prank, or challenge someone to wrestle.

202.
REFLECT
AND
RENEW

Use this review to make a list of five fun things
you want to do in the next few months!

Be it make homemade pasta, learn how to paint,
head off on a getaway with a friend, or learn
how to whistle – just make it fun.

203. **TWO-MINUTE WORKOUT: SUPERMAN UP AND AWAY!**

We all want some superpowers, right? Lie face down with arms and legs extended. Keeping the torso as still as possible, simultaneously raise the arms and legs to form a small curve in the body. Do this ten times, rest, and repeat. **Dani**

204. **WHAT RELAXES YOU?**

We all have our own ways of relaxing, but here's what often happens: as the time comes to spend some free time, we easily conform to the preferences of our partner, friend, or kids. We then wonder why we don't feel relaxed and recharged after. If you only do things that others want to do, and not what you need, then it's no wonder you're not feeling relaxed at the end of it. So do an activity that relaxes you!

205. **COIN COLLECTION**

Take ten minutes and collect all the loose change
you can find – from your bag, your wallet, your dresser,
and your coat pockets. Sort it, total it, and put it into bags
marked with the amount – and then spend it. It feels like
free money, and you'll be happier without all that loose
change rattling around. **Caroline**

206. **TWO-MINUTE WORKOUT: SQUAT WHILE YOU DO**

Squatting tones not only your glutes but your core and legs,
too. Record how many squats you can do in two minutes,
then try to beat your score each time. This is also great for
multitasking. For example, are you brushing your teeth or
waiting for the kettle to boil, or even waiting for the bus?
Squat while you do. **Dani**

207. **WHAT YOU LIKE ABOUT SOMEONE**

Choose a person close to you and identify one thing about
them that makes them special. Be it a personal trait, a skill,
or a passion, everyone has something that makes them
unique. What is it for that person? Write it down and –
for the best effect – tell them you appreciate it.

....

....

....

....

....

....

....

....

208. **A RELAXING SONG**

Music has been shown to have great powers over the
human mind. One of them is the ability to relax us. Listen to
a relaxing song. Lie down. Unwind. Let your thoughts drift.
You'll soon feel rested and at ease.

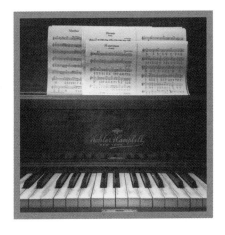

209. **FEET UP**

When you simply put your feet up, you are signaling to your body and mind that you are switching from an active state to resting. Just a small moment of relaxation with your feet up eases stress, enhances circulation, and relaxes you. As a bonus, it gives you a whole new perspective on your current surroundings. So put your feet up!

210. **PAUSE MINDFULLY**

Use a natural pause to practice some mindfulness. Don't wait impatiently for the green man at the crosswalk – use this as a chance to stop, breathe, and look around. Or if you're standing in a line, or boiling water, or pausing at work, just appreciate the moment.

211. **CELEBRATE COLOR**

We've all heard that blue makes you calm, yellow is the color of happiness, etc. The science on the psychology of color can be fluffy, but many of us still perceive its powers. So today, wear something colorful: add a splash of color to your home or office, find some color in nature, or put color on your plate. You could choose your favorite color, one to reflect your mood, or the best brain stimulus – try one you wouldn't normally choose and see how it makes you feel! **Tara**

212. **READ A POEM**

Reading poetry affects the brain in many of the same ways music does – it stimulates emotional and memory-related areas. Are you a poetry rookie? Give it a try today – you've got nothing to lose.

213. **FOOD, GLORIOUS FOOD**

You know I'm bonkers about food, and I want you to be, too.
For me, enjoying a delicious meal, made from scratch, with my
family, is the most beautiful thing. Simply appreciate your food
today. It could be a particularly mouthwatering ingredient,
the place you're eating in, the people you're with, or the
whole shebang! Simple, wonderful stuff. Enjoy. **Jamie**

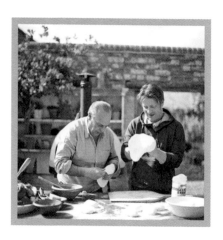

214. **SPOT A BEAUTIFUL BUILDING**

When we walk down the street we tend to keep our eyes fixed
either on the ground, on the ad-filled window displays, or, even
worse, glued to our smartphones – and we neglect to look up.
When walking down a familiar street, look up and
pay attention to the buildings. Take in the splendor of your
neighborhood architecture and try to select the most beautiful
building you see today.

215. **IMPROVE YOUR SLEEP ENVIRONMENT**

Sleep is one of the most important factors for our health,
but it's one of the first things we skimp on when work, family
life, or social life takes over. Better sleep is connected
to weight loss, stress reduction, and improved physical
performance. So buy a new pillow, make your bedroom
darker, use a different alarm clock, or cool down the room.
Whatever will get you to snooze better.

216. **GIVE A BOOK TO A FRIEND**

Good books are like portable magic, and we often have very personal relationships with our favorite books. Today, pick one book to give to a friend who you think might enjoy it. Discussing it later will not only deepen your bond but may provide new insights and new dimensions to the book that you have never thought about yourself.

217. **A PASSION OF YOURS**

What is a topic you feel really passionate about? We all have one (or a few) things that make our eyes twinkle, our minds start racing with ideas, and our excitement levels build – or that simply make us happy when we think about them. Be it gardening, BASE jumping, cooking, work, fashion, or collecting old car parts – spend a moment today reflecting on what it is for you and what you are doing to make it a part of your life.

218. TWO-MINUTE WORKOUT: SQUAT-TASTIC

The gluteus maximus is the biggest muscle in your body and it burns energy very quickly. Squats are a great way to activate your glutes and get your blood pumping. Rattle out ten squats – anytime, anywhere – to give yourself an energy boost. **Jamie S**

219. DRESS TO IMPRESS

What we wear can give us a major confidence boost. Today, wear something that you really like and that makes you look really good. Look good – feel great!

220. **HOW DO YOU FEEL TODAY?**

Be honest. How do you feel today? Worried? Inspired?
Excited? Happy? Expectant? Confused?

Write it down here and take a moment to reflect
on why you feel that way:

....

....

....

....

....

....

....

....

221. **VISIT A HIGH PLACE**

Today, climb, ride, or walk up to a high place. Not only is this a great way to exercise, but you may also get the chance to appreciate a stunning or interesting view. Use this as an opportunity to spend some time reflecting on your day.

222. **HIGH-FIVE YOURSELF**

Your most important relationship is to yourself – how you feel about yourself will color all of your relationships. Keeping a negative mental pattern about your shortcomings will keep the best you from the world. Jot down some really good things about you and what you've accomplished, and every time a negative thought enters your head today, drive it away by patting yourself on the back for one of your good qualities or achievements. You just might feel yourself soaring! **Caroline**

223. **TAKE A MICRO-BREAK**

Today, take a micro-break during the day. "Take a break!"
is not a popular thing to say to anyone who's really busy, but
even a brief timeout will make you more productive overall.
What does a micro-break look like for you today? Is it a cup of
tea alone, a walk around the office, taking a moment to look
out of the window, or simply turning your face to the sun?

224. **MORNING STRETCH**

After a night in bed, stretching is one of the best gifts you can
give your body. Gently wake up your muscles and joints –
stretch your arms, back, and legs first thing – and keep
yourself flexible. One minute is enough, and a great habit to
get into.

225. **THE MAGIC OF TOUCH**

Really tuning into our sense of touch can be one of the most amazing ways to practice mindfulness. Have you ever really stopped to think about how the fresh air feels on your skin? How real leather can feel both soft and rough? How a loved one's skin feels to the touch? Or how it feels to experience the warmth of a fire? Take a moment to mindfully tune into your sense of touch.

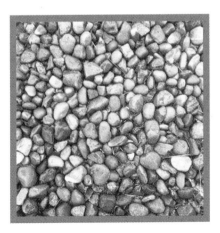

226. **DO SOMETHING YOU LOVED AS A KID**

Your memory is a very strong tool. Recalling good memories is
great for boosting your mood and happiness. The more details,
the better. So take a moment to recall your childhood joys.
And, even better, try to relive it!

....

....

....

....

....

....

....

....

....

227. **REARRANGE YOUR APPS**

What's front and center on your cell phone screen determines your phone habits and can affect your productivity. Move the most important features and apps to your home screen and arrange the apps you use less (or think you should use less!) in folders. You'll be surprised to find how easy access reduces stress and helps you to maintain focus. **Caroline**

228. **READ A WEBSITE RELATED TO YOUR JOB**

Take five minutes to explore a website related to your job or hobby. There could be interesting research on an industry website, new ideas on a competitor's site, or news and postings you weren't aware of. Keeping up-to-date with what's happening in your field will help generate new ideas – a core productivity activity. **Caroline**

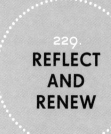

229.
REFLECT
AND
RENEW

Along any journey there are always rough patches.

Look back on the last year and identify one instance when you felt like you failed, couldn't go on, or had let yourself or someone else down.

Reflect on that situation and forgive yourself.

It's what's ahead that matters.

FOOD

230. **EPIC EGGS**

Inside each eggshell is an impressive nutrient arsenal.
The humble egg is packed with protein, and two eggs will
provide you with a source of a whopping eleven different
vitamins and minerals! Make eggs part of a meal today.
It still boggles my mind how affordable they are and how
many quick meals you can make with eggs, so whether you
fry, poach, scramble, boil, or whip up a frittata or omelette,
get cracking! Just remember to choose free-range or
organic if you can. **Jamie**

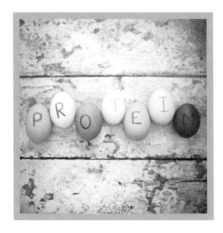

231. **EAT LUNCH AWAY FROM YOUR DESK**

Take thirty minutes to enjoy your lunch away from phone,
email, and other interruptions, and you'll likely have a more
productive afternoon. The break will allow you to savor your
meal, consider afternoon priorities, and come back to work
with renewed focus. **Caroline**

232. **YOUR FAVORITE MICRO-ACTION**

Which micro-action has been your favorite so far?
Take a moment to reflect on it, record it here, and repeat it.

....

....

....

233. **CLOSE YOUR EYES FOR A MINUTE**

Don't overthink your breaks. This time, just close your eyes
for one minute. Block out what's happening around you
and let your thoughts drift.

234. **TWO-MINUTE WORKOUT:**
LOW-SQUAT SITTING

Isometric exercises (holding a position) can be a pain in the
butt (literally), but they are great for building up your strength.
The low-squat position is the natural resting position for us
humans, and it's a great way to open up the hip area. So,
adopt the low-squat position and hold! See if you can
keep going for five minutes. **Jamie S**

235. **A RANDOM ACT OF KINDNESS**

Kindness makes us feel good – that's clear. But did you know
that kindness is also linked to happiness and health on a
biochemical level? Kindness causes the release of oxytocin
and dopamine in the brain, which contribute to reducing
inflammation in the body and can slow the aging process. Who
could you show a random act of kindness to today?

236. **YOUR PRODUCTIVITY TIP**

Productivity means efficiency (doing things faster or better)
but, above all, effectiveness (doing only the right things).
What helps you do your best work? How do you save time
in your daily routine? How do you prioritize a long to-do list?
Be creative, be practical, and inspire others with one
productivity tip that really works for you.

237. **JAZZ UP YOUR BREAKFAST**

Add a healthy twist to your breakfast today. Getting a good
dose of nutrients under your belt in the morning will really
set you up for the day ahead. So jazz up your breakfast with
a nutrient-packed twist. Add fresh fruit to your oatmeal,
have a dollop of natural yogurt on your cereal, swap butter for
avocado on your toast, or choose poached eggs over
fried. The key to keeping up good habits is to enjoy them,
so have fun and see what works for you. **Jamie**

238. **STIMULATE YOUR SENSES**

Today, really engage your senses. Walk barefoot,
eat a piece of dark chocolate, watch the sunset,
listen to the sea, try out some perfumes . . .
whatever you choose, enjoy it.

239. **BE MEDIOCRE – PROUDLY!**

It's wonderful to be brilliant at something. Most of the time, however, we're pretty mediocre. And that's good – if we accept it! Today, practice some self-acceptance and celebrate the mediocre. Enjoy a normal moment in your life, just as it is. Self-acceptance is an important driver for happiness and the ability to function well. Be perfectly imperfect and proud of it.

240. **MAKE A SEASONAL FILE**

You don't need to design a comprehensive filing system to be organized – one key file can make all the difference. This file labeled for the season will collect all those loose papers you need to keep for a while but not forever, such as receipts and bills. Put event tickets and vacation plans in the file, or an invite to a friend's party. When the season rolls around next year, go through the file and toss everything that's out of date. Easy and effective! **Caroline**

241. **SET THE TONE FOR THE WEEK**

"Start as you mean to go on" is a great mantra.
So today, set the tone for the week to come. Put a positive
spin on a problem, start the morning with a lovely breakfast,
complete a few small to-dos, decide on one important thing
you will get done, or simply smile brightly at someone.
What will your week look like?

....

....

....

....

....

....

....

....

242. **TWO-MINUTE WORKOUT: HOPPING**

Stand on one leg, hop for ten counts, then swap legs and repeat. Single-leg exercises engage smaller muscles in ways we can't duplicate when training both legs together. This translates into more balanced growth and development. **Dani**

243. **FINISH EATING BY 8 PM TONIGHT**

How does not eating late at night help improve productivity? You'll sleep better if you don't have food to digest sitting in your belly, and a good night's rest leads to a happier, more productive day. You'll also be more likely to eat a real breakfast tomorrow morning, setting you up for steady energy all day. One small change, many benefits. **Caroline**

244. **PLAN YOUR DREAM MORNING**

What is your favorite way to start a new day? Do you enjoy waking up a few minutes early? Doing some stretches? Maybe listening to a favorite song and eating a nutritious breakfast without distractions? Planning something that would make you really, really happy will help steer your thoughts and actions more than you might realize. So today, plan a dream morning that will properly set the tone of the day!

245. **TWO-MINUTE WORKOUT: VIRTUAL BIKE RIDING**

It's time to ride your virtual bicycle. Lie down with knees bent and hands behind your head. With your knees in toward your chest, bring your right elbow toward the left knee as the right leg straightens. Continue alternating sides (like you're pedaling). Just leave your helmet in the wardrobe. **Dani**

246. **TASTE IT**

For this micro-action, we'll turn food into a mindful moment.
We often rush through our meals. It's natural when we're in
a hurry, but we even tend to rush through the meals we have
time to enjoy. Today, when you eat, pick one thing you will really
savor. For example, take a tomato and cut it into pieces.
What's the texture? Where do you feel the taste in your mouth?
Is it sweeter or more savory than other tomatoes? How do the
seeds, skin, and pulp feel and taste? How long can you
enjoy that one tomato?

247. **DEFINE A REWARD FOR AN UNPLEASANT TASK**

No one wants to get down and dirty with unpleasant tasks.
Motivate yourself with a nice reward. It can be a piece of
chocolate, a bubble bath, or whatever puts a smile on your
face. Then do the task and get the reward!

248. **DRAW OR DOODLE SOMETHING**

Use this space to draw or doodle something small. How about the view out of the window, an object you see near you, a cartoon, or something you used to draw as a child? Don't worry about accuracy – the important thing is to let your creativity flow!

249. **DON'T DO SOMETHING**

Pick one thing you do habitually that hampers your productivity and give it a rest today. Your not-to-do item on this list might be "don't interrupt," "don't put myself down," "don't click on trashy celebrity stories" or "don't shop on the internet." See how you feel after you don't do it for one day. You'll be surprised how twenty-four hours can give you a new perspective. **Caroline**

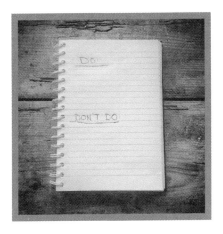

250. **GOOD ADVICE YOU'VE RECEIVED**

Recall one piece of good advice you've received in the past.
Something that made you stop and think, changed how you
look at life or at a specific problem. Was it an instant "Eureka!"
moment or did the advice inspire you over a longer period
of time? Share it today and maybe you can help
someone else in return.

....

....

....

....

....

....

....

....

251. **TACKLE A DIFFICULT CONVERSATION**

Whether it's a phone call you've been dreading or an uncomfortable work discussion, deferring a difficult conversation will depress your productivity all day. Tackle it first thing and see your output soar afterward. **Caroline**

252. **ENJOY A PUT-DOWN-FREE DAY**

Putting yourself and others down creates an atmosphere of negativity that can depress you and dampen productivity. For today, keep it all positive! Don't gossip about a friend, dismiss a colleague's idea, or tell your children that their friends have better manners. And be kind to yourself, too – say only positive things about yourself for twenty-four hours. Feel your can-do coming on? **Caroline**

253. **TWO-MINUTE WORKOUT: KNEE LIFTS**

Standing with your feet hip-width apart, lift one leg up toward your chest as high as you can and lower it back down to the ground. Repeat with your other leg. Standing knee lifts are great for boosting strength in your midsection as they don't isolate the abdominal muscles in the way that standard crunches do. Instead, they work your abs in conjunction with other key muscles. **Dani**

254. **ACT HOW YOU WANT TO FEEL**

The link between mind and body is tremendous. Today, make your body act the way you want to feel. When you feel tired your posture worsens, but this is true in the reverse as well. Smile and you'll feel happier. Stand in a power position and you'll feel more confident. Physically reach out to someone and you'll feel more connected. Acting on this insight can truly be one of the greatest changes in your life.

LOVE

255. **DREAM AWAY**

Today, take a moment to daydream. Studies have demonstrated that the brain solves tough problems in the background while daydreaming. So those brilliant ideas or epiphany moments don't just "come to you," they are the by-product of unconscious mental activity when your brain is resting. Feed your brain by giving it some downtime and daydream away.

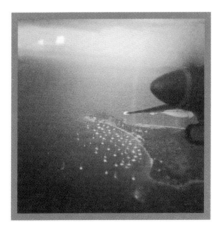

256. **LONG-DISTANCE LOVING**

Sometimes we've all got to be reminded to do something nice
for someone we love who's not always around – whether it's
your mom, dad, aunt, mentor, or your best friend who's moved
out of town. Today, surprise someone you don't often see
and remind them how much you love them and why.

257. **CLEAN A SURFACE**

Today, at home or at work, zero in on an appliance, cupboard,
light fixture, shelf, table, or windowsill that's not on your
sponge's daily circuit and give it a minute of cleaning.
It will give the whole room a lift and prove that finding
time just means finding a minute. **Caroline**

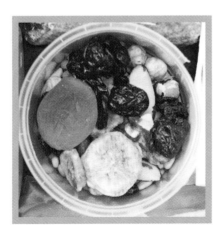

258. **PREPARE A SNACK**

To tackle the snack attack, pack or prep a healthy snack.
We've all been there, caught off guard by hunger pangs
and impulsively grabbing the nearest (often not-so-healthy!)
nibble. So today, get ahead and be ready for the snack
attack – throw a small handful of nuts and dried fruit in a
container, pack some crunchy veggie sticks with a little
hummus, or simply toss an apple in your bag before
you head out of the door. **Jamie**

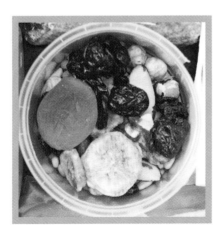

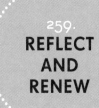

259.
REFLECT
AND
RENEW

Take a moment to reflect on the micro-actions
you've undertaken over the last month.

What have you achieved?

About which areas of your life are you
feeling particularly positive?

Are there things you feel you can improve on?

260. **RUN UP THE STAIRS**

Today, ban the elevator and use the stairs. Stepping is a great
way to get the heart pumping, especially on the way into work,
before and after lunch, and on the way home. Use the stairs
today for that extra burst of energy. Try to find a place where
you can run up at least five flights of stairs. **Jamie S**

261. **EXTEND YOUR NETWORK**

Building networks increases productivity by enabling us to
access advice, referrals, and administrative shortcuts. Visit the
desk of a colleague or ask out a fledgling connection for a quick
cup of coffee. It only takes ten minutes to build a bridge.
Caroline

262. **TECH TIMEOUT**

Deep down, many of us know we're a bit addicted to technology and too contactable. For your own benefit, it's good to draw some clear tech rules. How will you take a tech timeout today and what are your tech-timeout rules?

....

....

263. **SMILE AT A STRANGER**

Has someone ever suddenly smiled at you on a busy street? Do you remember the feeling after the initial surprise? Today, when you are out and about, smile at a stranger. Smiling will make you feel happier and more confident for reaching out to others.

FOOD

264. **A HEALTHY MEAL**

We often start our diets and lifestyle improvements with drastic measures and overnight changes. But many times you don't need to change up everything to eat healthier (it can even make you more likely to fall off the wagon) – just make some improvements here and there. Have one meal you consider healthy today. Be it a balanced breakfast, lunch with a side salad, a smart snack to keep the cravings at bay, or a veggie-heavy dinner. How do you eat healthier? One meal at a time.

LOVE

265. **GIVE SOMEONE A GIFT**

Have you ever received a small gift unexpectedly? How did that feel? No need to wait for birthdays, Christmas, or anniversaries – the best time to give a gift is today. It doesn't need to be big – send a postcard, pick up some flowers, get those favorite chocolates, or simply do something you know will make another person happy.

266. **SET YOUR ALARM CLOCK FOR AN EARLIER START**

Set your alarm clock thirty minutes earlier for tomorrow. Plan
one thing you'll do in the morning with that extra time.
Will you read, take a walk, use the time for creative writing,
or maybe just sit on the balcony and admire the view?
These micro-pockets of "extra" time can sometimes
be the most valuable.

267. **A GREEN MO(VE)MENT**

Put on your walking shoes and head out. Combine a moment
of natural wonderment with some light exercise. What does
nature look like where you are and how are you making
the most of it? You don't need much – just five minutes of
"green exercise" can improve your mood and self-esteem.

268. **TRY A NEW THING**

We often get stuck in our routines and, while routines give great structure to the day, it's good to mix things up occasionally and explore the new. So cycle along a different route, try a new sport, shop for food in a new place, wear a color you usually don't, sign up to learn something, test a new type of drink, or simply try looking at the world in a different way. Try one new thing today.

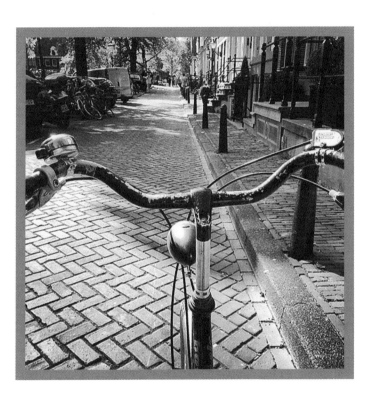

269. **TAKE AN INTEREST**

Is there a person in your life who goes on about a particular project, hobby, or sport with a fervor you don't feel? Instead of trying to avoid the subject or slip away, change it up by prompting your enthusiast to tell you all about it – and listen! Take this opportunity to prompt a partner, friend, or family member to tell you about their favorite topic while you give them your best attention. You're going to create some really good vibes! **Caroline**

270. **BANISH THE MONDAY BLUES**

Come Monday morning, many of us feel the "Monday blues." Don't let them define your week! Today, do, experience, think of, or invent something to cheer you up and banish those Monday blues.

271. **MAKE A DECISION**

Often we do not only procrastinate about to-dos but also about decisions. An unmade decision can lurk in the back of your mind and cause you stress without you even realizing it – and vice versa: making a decision can release energy and steer you in a desired direction. So today, make one small decision – something you've been putting off – or simply decide quickly on one thing you're presented with. Holiday plans, a small purchase decision, or something bigger like a shift in career – be brave!

272. **PLATE IT**

It's easy to lose track of food and eat mindlessly when you're eating directly out of a bag or box. For both meals and snacks it helps to see exactly how much you will be eating before you start, which creates a natural boundary to how much you eat. Put everything you plan to eat on a plate before enjoying it. **Darya**

273. **FIND BEAUTY AROUND YOU**

Take a moment to notice the beauty all around you.
There's beauty on every street corner, in every home and
office cubicle, and in that person sitting opposite you.
Focus on the moment and give it your full attention.

274. **ENJOY YOUR FAVORITE TUNES**

Music distracts the mind and induces a state of calmness.
It slows your heart rate and breathing, lowers blood pressure,
and reduces the stress hormone norepinephrine, which is
associated with insomnia. Take a moment to listen to some
of your favorite music today.

FOOD

275. SIP YOUR DRINK

Taking sips of water or another drink regularly throughout your meal can help you slow down and remember to chew as you eat. A bonus is you'll get extra hydration and fill up faster. What are you drinking today? **Darya**

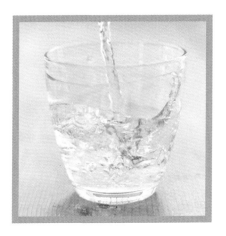

276. **AN ACTIVITY THAT BRINGS JOY**

Sometimes exercise can feel like a drag! It can seem big, scary, and time-consuming – difficult to even get started. So today, make movement a happy thing and do something that brings you joy. What activity is the most joyful for you? **Jamie S**

277. **WHAT HAVE YOU DONE FOR YOU TODAY?**

This is a simple question, yet one we should all answer at the end of each day. Do your days get filled up with chores, work, meetings, and helping others? It's important not only to take "me time," but also to think about it as a necessity – not an occasional luxury. So what have you consciously done today just for you? Meditate, eat your vitamins, read a book, sit down with a cup of coffee, spend time with your coloring book, or take a warm bath.

278. **READ A SUMMARY OF TODAY'S NEWS**

Expanding our awareness of current affairs helps us gain
perspective beyond our own lives. Today, read a summary
of the news. What stands out? What makes you think?

279. **A PRESENT YOU WANT**

At some point during this year it will be your birthday,
and whether you're a fan of birthdays or not, it's a good
day to pause and reflect. This year, focus on yourself –
decide one thing you will do for you. Get yourself a present
no one knows you want, book in some "me" time, or treat
yourself to something.

280. **SORT YOUR MAIL**

Take a moment when you pick up your mail to toss all
the junk and to open routine items. You'll be surprised how
manageable that stack of letters becomes if you throw flyers,
circulars, and unwanted magazines away immediately.
Caroline

281. **MOVE IN A NEW WAY**

Whether you take a class, break into dance, or go for a walk,
hike, jog, bike ride, or skate – moving doesn't have to be about
pain and sweat. The more variety the better for your body, and
you won't get bored. Today, pick something active you've not
tried before and move in a new way. **Jamie S**

282. **CONSIDER THE DAY AHEAD**

Either you run the day or the day runs you. Sit down for
a moment and walk through your day. What is important?
What is not? What do you want to achieve? Then do it.

Make a plan here:

....

....

....

....

....

....

....

....

283. **CELEBRATE SALAD**

Make salad part of a meal today or, even better, the main
event. The possibilities are endless: warm, cold, chopped,
shaved, leafy, meaty, hearty, light . . . I could go on!
Have fun mixing up flavors, textures, and great combos.
You might go for a hearty main, a sexy side salad, or
a killer sandwich filling. Over to you. **Jamie**

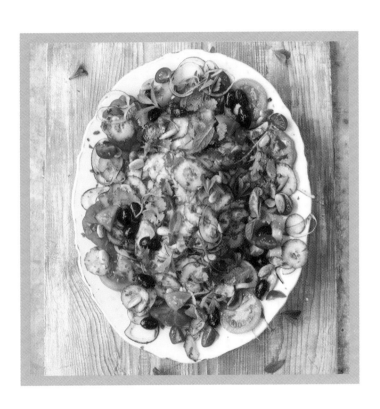

284. **A SMALL SOCIAL MEDIA CHANGE**

Today, make one small social media change that supports
your happiness. At best, social media enhances our
relationships with other people and freshens our thinking,
but it can also make us unhappy, addicted, and restless.
By being more aware of how we want to use social media,
we can gain more well-being from it. Today, make one small,
positive change in the way you use social media. Replace
social media time with some other worthwhile activity;
unfollow pages or users that you no longer want to follow;
send a nice message to a friend you haven't been in touch
with for a while; or spread something valuable, like positivity,
compassion, or an interesting article in a post.

285. **DIM THE LIGHTS**

Optimize your environment for mindful eating by lighting
a candle or dimming the lights. Research has shown
you eat faster under bright light, so set the mood
and enjoy the change of pace. **Darya**

286. **BEST PART OF YOUR DAY**

Mindfulness is often about being present in small moments.
Today, capture a moment that you enjoyed, however
simple, and record it here:

....

....

....

....

....

....

....

....

....

....

287.
REFLECT
AND
RENEW

Throughout the course of this book, you've hopefully been forming some sustainable habits that will last you the rest of your life.

Make a list of the things that have become a habit and celebrate them!

LOVE

288. **ACCEPT YOURSELF**

Such a cliché, but it's true: you are the most important person
in your life. Accept yourself with all your quirks and "flaws"
today. Do something to treat yourself – you deserve it.

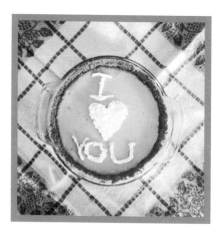

289. **RECALL SOMETHING FUNNY**

Overwhelming day? Do you have a lot on your plate right now?
Remembering fun things tickles the pleasure center of the brain
and helps you relax. So recall a fun memory, a good
joke, or something that made you smile.

290. **SORT YOUR PHONE PHOTOS**

Never has snapping a pic been easier or less expensive. But
our ongoing personal documentaries take up a lot of digital
space, and finding the really memorable photos can be a hunt.
Take five minutes and scan recent photos. Of your last thirty
selfies, how many do you really want to keep? What about
photos of meals or a coat in a window you admired? Clearing
out photos will free up space on your phone but also distill your
snapshots into something more memorable. **Caroline**

291. **TAKE A MOMENT IN NATURE**

Today, take a moment to go out and enjoy nature.
Do you see budding spring flowers? Or the first signs
of autumn? Just five minutes of active time outside is
good for your mood and self-esteem, so get out there.

292. **ORGANIZE YOUR CLOTHES FOR TOMORROW**

Lay out what you will wear tomorrow, right down to the tie,
tights, earrings, or cuff links. Get it done early, before you are
so wiped out that you can't be bothered. You'll sleep better
and longer knowing that you won't be hunting down a shoe
or hastily redressing when you discover too late that you're
missing a button or that your shirt has a stain. **Caroline**

293. **SOMETHING TO LOOK FORWARD TO**

Anticipating future fun is an easy way to improve your mood and broaden your perspective from the daily routine. Put on your adventure hat and plan a getaway, a special event, a night out, or an exciting change in your life. What are you looking forward to?

294. **CLEAR OUT FIVE ITEMS**

Reorganizing your desk, kitchen, files, and drawers is usually on everyone's to-do list but seldom gets addressed. Half the battle is weeding out items of minimal (or negative) utility. Open a drawer today and challenge yourself to get rid of at least five things. **Caroline**

295. DO A TASK YOU'VE BEEN PUTTING OFF

Select one task languishing on your to-do list. Pick up that extension cord at the DIY shop, change the hard-to-reach light bulb in that closet, call an elderly relative, make an appointment to get your teeth checked. Pick one thing from your nagging to-do list and get it done today. **Caroline**

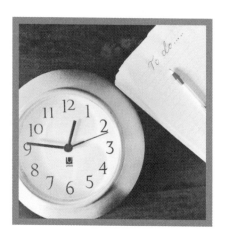

296. **A MINDFUL WALK**

Walking mindfully can have an amazing, calming effect. Try walking in sync with your body and with nature. Begin by becoming aware of how your body feels. What is your posture like? How about your breathing? Are they changing during your walk? Then, switch your focus to the surroundings: What sounds can you hear? What is the wind like today? Have your surroundings changed since you were last there?

297. **CUDDLE AN ANIMAL**

Time spent with animals is a guaranteed happiness boost – hospitals and nursing homes often practice animal therapy for precisely this reason. Being with our furry friends simply gives us a feeling of well-being. So cuddle your pet, your neighbor's cat, or take a walk to the nearest park to get your dose of animal love.

298. **DO YOUR BIT TO SAVE WATER**

Have your daily dose to drink, but also do one small micro-action to reduce your water consumption. Fix a leak, turn off the tap while brushing your teeth, use less water for the dishes, don't dwell in the shower. You can also save water in less obvious ways. Did you know that 2½ gallons of water are used to make one sheet of paper, and 24 gallons are used to make 1 pound of plastic? Could you cut some out from your life?

299. **TAKE THE STAIRS AFTER LUNCH**

After your lunch today, climb a flight or two of stairs. Instead of taking the elevator back to your office, walk up part of the way. If you ate at your desk, walk down a flight or two and then come back. Simple exertion will help jump-start your metabolism just when digestion is slowing it down and help you have a productive afternoon. **Caroline**

300. **CLOSE YOUR EYES**

Take a few minutes and simply close your eyes. Set a timer and take a comfortable position – sitting in a chair, outside on a park bench, or laying down on the floor or sofa. Just relax for a moment. A great micro-action to find your "Zen" at any point during the day!

301. **A MAN YOU ADMIRE**

Today, consider which man in your life you look up to and why. Is it your dad, grandfather, friend, neighbor, a teacher, or someone else who has left a positive mark on your life? Reflect on him today.

FOOD

302. **FISH MISSION**

Try a fish you've never had before. There are so many species of fish out there, yet we tend to stick to just a handful of varieties. In the US, it's usually tuna, salmon, and tilapia. They may be delicious, but there are a lot of alternatives, and choosing a different fish not only means we can help relieve overfished and threatened species, but also that we discover new flavors to fall in love with. Speak to your fishmonger, see what they recommend, and go fish! Choose responsibly sourced options, if you can. **Jamie**

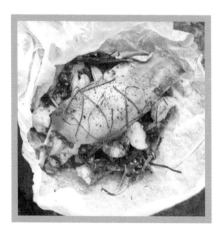

303. **DANCE LIKE NO ONE'S WATCHING**

Moving your body is an incredible thing, especially when
you can rock it to your favorite tunes. So get moving today –
be it in the car, on your way to work, at home, or in the office.
Turn it up and dance for the entire song! **Dani**

304. **PICK UP A CLASSIC**

Books have the unique ability to take us on a journey
through space, time, perspective, and reality. The classics
may feel dry and antiquated, but they have stood the test
of time and can be surprisingly relevant to us now, even
when written hundreds of years ago. Pick up a classic
book you want to read or have read before and loved –
and see where it takes you.

FOOD

305. **HANDY HYDRATION**

Today, keep water handy. I've talked about it before, but it's important to repeat to get into the habit. Two-thirds of our bodies are made up of water, so if you're not hydrated, you're not at your best. Wherever you are, make it easy to refill with humble H_2O. Stash a bottle in your bag, keep a glass filled at your desk, and pop a jug on the dinner table. The beauty of water is that it's so simple and cheap to hydrate – all you have to do is turn on the tap. Bottoms up! **Jamie**

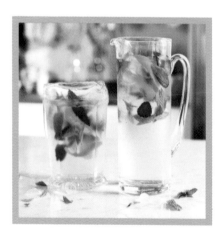

306. **GO BAREFOOT**

We spend so much time in socks or shoes. Today, take yours off and go barefoot, even just at home. For the best experience, go outside and walk on fresh grass, and really feel the ground under the soles of your feet.

307. **LIGHT A CANDLE**

Candles are magical and powerful things. They bring light to the darkness and warmth to the cold. Light a candle today and remember a loved one, celebrate a special day, embrace a moment of quietness, or simply just enjoy the soft atmosphere it creates.

308. **WALK, EVERY HOUR, ON THE HOUR**

Today, set your alarm to ring every hour. When the alarm goes off, get up and walk around. No need to make it a long walk – even just around the room is enough to be beneficial. **Jamie S**

309. **MAKE A BETTER CHOICE**

Make one choice a better one. We make thousands of choices every day, and research says we're unconscious of as many as 60 percent of those. We run on autopilot and repeat the same things from one day to the next. It's really the small changes we make here and there that truly make a difference. So make a better choice. Today, have a healthier breakfast, lay out your running gear in the evening to get you motivated in the morning, spend some time outside, or work standing up for a bit.

310. **WRITE DOWN A THOUGHT**

What's one thing you have on your mind right now? Is it an undone task that keeps bugging you? A nice event you're looking forward to? A feeling you have but cannot fully comprehend or express? Writing it down focuses your thinking. This can also give your mind a break and the thing itself a bit more perspective. So pick up your pen and do your best to express it in words here:

....

....

....

....

....

....

....

311. **DAILY DAIRY**

Unless you're a vegan or intolerant, dairy is an important part of your diet. Make sure you include a little bit of dairy in a meal today. As well as being a great source of calcium and vitamin A, dairy foods are packed with protein, which is essential for growth and repair. It's true that some dairy products are also high in fat but, enjoyed in moderation, they have many benefits. Try adding a dollop of yogurt to a meal, finishing a dish with a grating of Parmesan, or embracing naturally lower-fat cheese choices such as feta, ricotta, or cottage cheese. **Jamie**

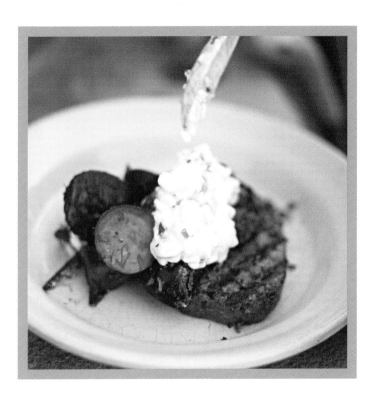

312. DON'T SUPERSIZE

Portion control for many of us has gone crazy. We're all guilty of sometimes going back for seconds (even thirds!) or happily devouring a large portion just because we're offered one. Today, pay attention when you portion your food. Don't pile your plate too high and be mindful of recommended serving sizes for things like pasta and rice – it sounds obvious, but if you measure it out before cooking, there'll be no leftovers to tempt you! **Jamie**

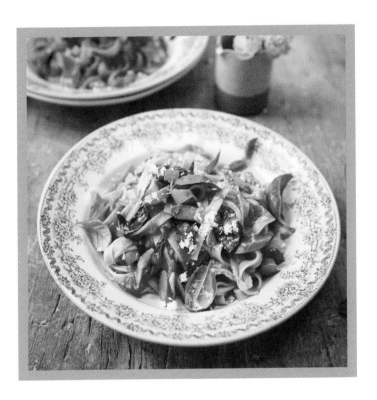

313. **TALK TO AN OLDER PERSON**

We often get caught in the here and now. As we grow older
we start seeing the patterns and the deeper meaning in life.
Gain perspective early – talk to an older person today.

314. **SHORTEN YOUR MEETINGS**

End hour-long meetings at fifty minutes; half hour ones at
twenty-five. If it's not your meeting, help it to end promptly once
its purpose has been accomplished. That extra ten minutes in
every hour will be a productivity boost for everyone involved.
Meeting adjourned. **Caroline**

315. **WRITE DOWN WHAT HAPPENED TODAY**

In the evening our brain is overloaded with stimuli from the day, which can make it hard to relax. Take a moment to write down the things on your mind from today. Then forget about them for tonight and have some downtime.

316. **BUILD UP AN APPETITE**

There's nothing like sitting down at the table with a big appetite, ready to dig in. Those amazing smells that make your mouth water and the feeling of satisfaction after a well-earned meal are hard to beat. Today, make an effort to build up an appetite, whether that means avoiding grazing, getting outside and active before sitting down, or simply waiting until you're truly hungry before having a meal. **Jamie**

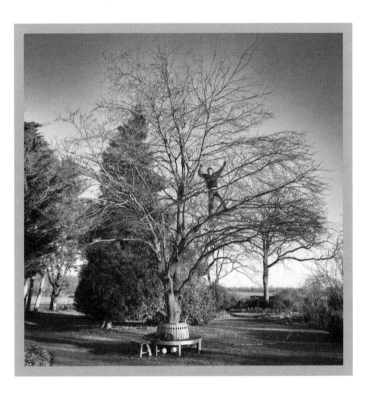

317.
REFLECT
AND
RENEW

We are nearing the end of this book and you've
now done more than 300 micro-actions for
a happier, healthier you.

Take a moment to look through your notes and start
forming a story of the person you are becoming.
Then share that story with someone – a friend,
partner, or family member. No doubt they'll be
happy to take part in it and help you forward.

318. **LOOK UP**

Today – simply look up. When we walk down familiar streets we tend to look down at the road or at our feet (or worse, our smartphones!). Yet, there are so many things to see if we change our perspective just a tiny bit, and by far the easiest way to do that is to simply look up. What do you see? A blue sky, approaching rain clouds, a nice balcony where someone is enjoying the day, or maybe you notice that the trees are changing color with the season.

319. **DO SOME PEOPLE WATCHING**

Every person who walks past you on the street or sits on the same bus as you has their own story. They have their dreams, fears, insecurities, victories, strengths, reasons to smile, and reasons to cry. Sit down today in a place with people around you and do some people watching. Try to construct the stories of those you see – their backgrounds, professions, highs and lows. It can really change the way you look at others.

320. **TOP 3 TODAY**

According to research, practicing gratitude regularly is one of the easiest and most "foolproof" actions to increase your happiness, by far. So write down the top three things that happened to you today. Was it time spent with someone important to you? A small success at work? An engaging discussion? A great meal? Or maybe a nice view along your walk?

321. **SPEND LESS ON SOMETHING**

Saving money depends as much upon small daily behaviors as conscious financial goal setting. Small spending decisions on coffees, magazines, lunch, taxi rides, and cocktails invisibly raise our daily expenses until we compromise our financial goals. Pick a situation and choose the less expensive choice: make your lunch, walk instead of taking the bus, or sip a glass of water instead of a martini. If you can make small cuts here and there, your wallet will thank you very soon. **Caroline**

FOOD

322. NATURALLY SWEET

Whether you have a sweet tooth or not, sugar usually plays a part in our day-to-day diets. We all know too much is bad for us, so minimize your processed-sugar intake today by sweetening your food and drinks with something natural. Try adding fruit to your breakfast instead of sugar, or using fresh fruit to flavor water rather than choosing a sugary drink. **Jamie**

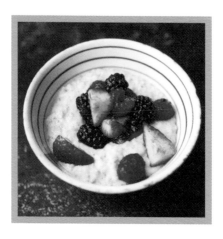

323. **YOUR GROWTH MOMENT**

Today, recall a moment of growth in your life. How has it
changed you or improved things for you? What did you learn?

Write it here:

....

....

....

....

....

....

....

....

....

324. SOMETHING YOU ALWAYS WANTED TO ASK

Children ask questions all the time. Often they ask questions we have never thought of, and we learn something new in the process. Today, ask a question you always wanted to know the answer to – you might be surprised at the answer.

325. DO ONE THING DIFFERENTLY

Routines and habits are comfortable and often desired. So challenge yourself once in a while. Change one thing. It might be big or small, related to movement, food, yourself, or the people you care about. Doing that one thing differently will stimulate your brain in new ways.

326. **BOOK A DATE WITH YOURSELF**

Think for a minute about the time and effort we put into treating the object of our affection when we go on a date, and how good that feels – for both parties! So why not extend that to yourself? Plan to take some time just for you – treat yourself to a movie, a glass of wine, a massage, or a walk. Or simply do something silly when you're home alone and no one is watching. Make it count for you!

327. **ORGANIZE YOUR CLOSET IN FIVE MINUTES**

Set a timer for five minutes and see how many items you can pull together in your closet to make it easier to find what you need. In this time, can you hang all your tops/shirts together in a group, line your shoes together in pairs, or remove any old plastic wrap and wire hangers from the rail? You can accomplish a lot in five minutes, and your next encounter with your closet will be quicker and more satisfying. **Caroline**

328. **REARRANGE A ROOM**

Do you dream about a complete room makeover but never quite achieve it? Making just one or two positive alterations can give you a real lift. Change it up whenever you've got ten minutes to spare. Move a lamp, hang a picture . . . and wouldn't that chair be better by the window? It's fun, it's fast, and it lasts. **Caroline**

329. **A WEAKNESS OF YOURS**

What is one weakness you have? Try to identify something you honestly want to work on and apply the "strength-based" approach to it. How can you use one of your strengths to help you improve on your weakness? For example, can you use your strength in planning to overcome your shyness in social situations?

330. **MAKE A RESOLUTION FOR TODAY**

When you make a specific resolution, you are up to ten times
more likely to keep it than if you have an unspecific goal.
Go ahead: make a resolution for something you will
do or achieve today. Write it here:

....

....

....

....

....

....

....

....

....

FOOD

331. **GO THE WHOLE WAY**

I've challenged you on this before. Quite simply, if you swap out white refined bread, pasta, rice, or noodles for the whole wheat or whole grain alternatives, it could be the easiest but biggest, most positive change you make to your diet this year. You'll get more depth of flavor, and as they're packed with fiber they'll keep you feeling fuller for longer, as well as help to lower blood cholesterol. **Jamie**

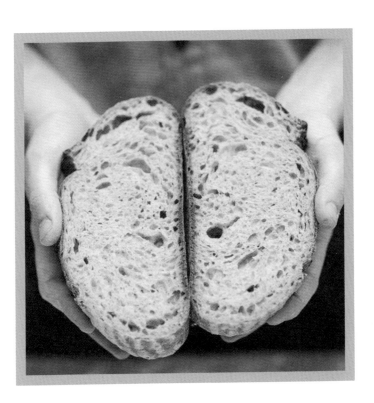

332. **FIND A NEW PLACE**

Today, take a mindful walk around your neighborhood and find
a new spot. Most days we walk the same streets and visit the
same places but do not really pay attention. Today, pick
up your coffee from somewhere else, have lunch in a different
location, pop into that bookshop you always wanted to visit,
or walk down a new road in your neighborhood or a path out
in the countryside. You may discover a new favorite place.

333. **GO PANTRY SHOPPING**

We all have those shadowy kitchen shelves filled with tins
and odds and ends. This micro-action is super simple. Root
around in a kitchen cabinet and use up one ingredient
rather than buying a duplicate you don't need. Next time
you go shopping to stock up on new items, check your
cabinets first for forgotten-about ingredients. We often fill
our shopping carts with things we already have, so you'll
reduce waste and save money – and you may even
uncover a tasty surprise! **Jamie**

334. MICRO-HELP SOMEONE

Today, micro-help someone else. Do a small deed,
show gratitude, say "thank you," offer a helping hand –
it'll be more than worth it.

335. WANDER AROUND

For today's lunch (or coffee break) go wander. Leave
the house or workplace and meander around the same way
you would if you were on vacation in a new place. Stroll
through the little park a few blocks away, window shop, or
browse in a bookstore. Research shows that environmental
stimulation helps us to maintain focus and mental energy.
Fifteen minutes will do the trick! **Caroline**

336. CALCULATE SOMETHING IN YOUR HEAD

Remember when you learned the multiplication tables by heart in school? How well can you do it now? Calculating simple things in your head is a skill you easily lose if you don't practice it. Try and do some mental math today.

337. TWO-MINUTE WORKOUT: BALANCE!

Proprioception (difficult word, I know!) is the body's ability to know its own position. Cues from the environment, your feet, inner ear, and eyes tell your body which muscles to use. Good balance means better coordination and posture. To train your balance, practice standing on one leg for two minutes. **Jamie S**

338. **WHAT MAKES YOU PROUD?**

What lifts your spirits? It could be something you did,
that someone else did, or something that you just think
is awesome in the world. Being able to enjoy the
"small things" will enable you to think positive.

Jot them down here:

339. **SPREAD POSITIVE ENERGY**

Remember that time when a stranger's smile made you smile as well? Or when a friend complimented you at just the right moment, and the course of your day changed in an instant? Every single encounter contains a possibility to choose what kind of energy we spread around us. A kind gesture of opening a door, chatting with the cashier, or sending a message to a friend can make the other person's day a bit happier — and it adds more positive seconds into your day as well!

340. **WASH FINGERPRINTS OFF A WALL**

Arm yourself with a soapy sponge or a spray cleaner and pick a wall or windowsill that needs attention, then go at it. You'll be surprised at how gratifying the result of five minutes' work can be. Try the areas around light switches for speedy satisfaction — they often get a bit grimy but clean up fast.

Caroline

341. **PUT ONE THING IN ITS PLACE**

Start the day organized. Choose one thing to pick up
and put in its place. Be it work papers, a pile of clothes,
or the children's toys – you've already achieved one
good thing today.

342. **CARRY YOUR WEIGHT**

At the supermarket? Pick a basket instead of a cart or,
even better, leave the car at home and walk to the store, and
carry your shopping bag. Muscles will have to work harder to
carry extra weight, which in turn will boost your metabolism,
strength, and circulation; improve core muscles; and give your
whole body a workout. **Jamie S**

343. **HELP SOMEONE OUT**

Who could you help today? We've all had those occasions in the past when someone has offered us a helping hand at the right moment. In many cases the feeling of helping, of giving without the need to get something in return, is an even better one. Provide a little help to someone today – a friend, neighbor, colleague, or a stranger on the street.

344. **SCHEDULE "ME" TIME**

Today, consciously put aside a bit of time for yourself. Many of us spend a lot of our time catering to other people's needs or doing what is expected of us. What would you do today if you could do anything, just for you? Schedule it in and take that time.

345. **READ SOMETHING POETIC**

Today, pick up a book or a poem and immerse yourself in
it for a moment. Whether you enjoy poetry or not, reading it
is one of the best ways to focus and stimulate your brain.
Poetry is an unexplored area for many, but the right poem
can whisk you away to another world.

346. **AN IMPORTANT MOMENT THIS WEEK**

Stopping to think about what has happened during the past
week can be very useful: we can learn to identify decisions and
actions that have been good for us, and then make more of
those next week. Also, reliving good moments doubles the joy!
So, today, think of a moment that was significant this week.
Was it a calming jog after work to help you relax? A nice dinner
with loved ones? A helpful meeting at work? Or maybe an
important realization?

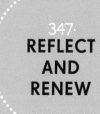

347.
**REFLECT
AND
RENEW**

For this review – take a moment and look back on your journey so far.

What changes are you seeing in yourself?

In what situations are you feeling the happiest, most accomplished, most self-assured?

How can you strengthen this feeling in yourself?

348. **VEGGIE BREAKFAST**

Mix things up today and incorporate a vegetable element into your breakfast. Variety is key for a healthy diet, and if you can get one of your five-a-day portions in your first meal, then you'll be off to a great start! Think creamy avocado on toast, fluffy sweet corn pancakes, a refreshing green smoothie, or a veg-packed omelet. **Jamie**

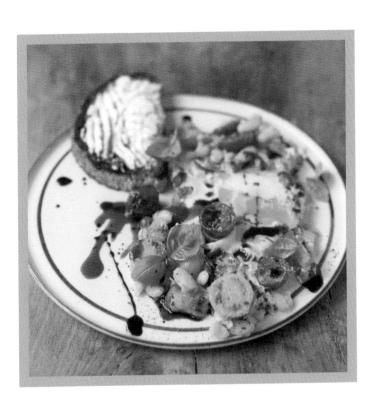

349. **CLEAR OUT YOUR UNDERWEAR DRAWER**

Nothing gets worn and washed as much as underwear, and there's a tendency to add new to old without really tossing out the truly tattered unmentionables. Take a moment to toss holey and unpaired socks, greyed-out camisoles, and elastic-less underwear. Even undercover, worn-out undies are a downer. **Caroline**

350. **REACH FOR THE FURTHEST PACKET**

Save on food waste – and hopefully save yourself a bit of cash, too. Reach to the back of one of your lesser-used cabinets and pick out a tin or packet to use up in a meal. Even though pantry items may feel like they last forever, you'll be surprised how many we let expire hiding away in the back. **Jamie**

351. WHO INSPIRES YOU?

It is human nature to search for answers to life's big questions,
and many of us do so by seeking inspiration from wise women
and men, past and present. Who is that person who inspires
you, makes you think, and, above all, would make you act?
Alive or long gone, famous or known by few, a specific person
or a group, think about how they inspire you today.

352. PAUSE YOUR MOVEMENT

Next time you're up and moving, pause your movement for just
two minutes. Moving your body every day is paramount for your
health, but so is taking breaks – it's when your muscles rest
and develop, and it can put you in touch with how your body is
feeling. How could you stop moving for two minutes? Cool
down after a workout, listen to a song, or take a stretching
break. Or, simply find a space where you can sit or lie down
and allow your body to relax. **Dani**

353. **REARRANGE YOUR WALLET**

Wallet full of old receipts? Still have foreign currency rattling around from your vacation nine months ago? How about all those business cards you intended to enter as contacts? Take five minutes today to rearrange your wallet: remove old papers, make the most important cards easily accessible, and get rid of change. You'll be surprised how much more rapid and stress-free your daily transactions will be after just a few small changes. **Caroline**

354. **LAY OUT YOUR WORKOUT CLOTHES**

A morning workout is a great habit to get into, but it can be really hard to get started. A simple way to give you that extra push is to lay out your exercise clothes right next to your bed the night before. It'll feel easier and more motivating in the morning, for sure.

355. **BEST OF THE YEAR**

Introspective thinking and writing can have numerous
health benefits. Today, look back at the past year.
What do you remember? What was the best, coolest,
funniest, most memorable part of the year gone by?
Was there something that you really loved?

Take a moment to record it here:

356. **ONE NEW FOOD SKILL**

Whether you teach yourself or someone else – get in the kitchen, try something new, and teach one food skill today. Learning a food skill is powerful and will stick with you for life, especially for kids, so if you have little ones in your life teach them something simple, such as how to make a salad dressing. Maybe you've always wanted to learn how to poach eggs perfectly or devein a juicy prawn. Whatever it is, give it a try! **Jamie**

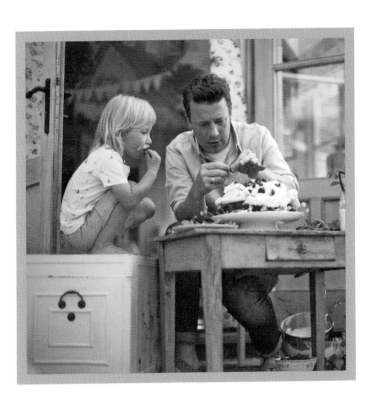

357. **WHAT MATTERS MORE THAN MONEY?**

Reflect on one thing that is more important to you than money. Money for many of us is important and can bring lots of opportunities. But if you think money will bring happiness, think again. Money is good, but many other things are better. If you had no wealth (or all the wealth in the world) what would matter most to you?

358. **SEND SNAIL MAIL**

In this day of electronic everything, we rarely turn to traditional "snail mail" (except for paper ads and bills). Today, make the mail carrier happy and send someone a letter or a postcard via traditional mail routes. Get a kick from imagining the joy and surprise of the person at the other end receiving your note!

359. **MORNING GLORY**

Whether you're a morning person or not, what happens in the first hour after waking up can have an immense impact on the rest of your day. Look back to micro-action 72: Modify One Morning Habit. What did you decide to change back then? If you're still sticking to it, maybe it's time to add another positive change. And if you're not sticking to it, try again or attempt a different one. Is eating breakfast your weak spot? Are you perpetually late in the morning? What could make your mornings go more smoothly?

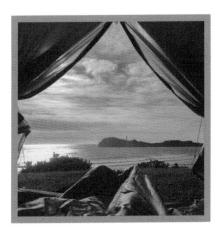

360. WHAT MAKES YOU ANGRY?

Anger is powerful. Anger can trigger the body's "fight or flight" response and be bad for your health, so it's a good idea to let off steam. Spend a few moments writing down what makes your blood boil. Then take a deep breath and let it go . . .

....

....

....

....

....

....

....

....

FOOD

361. **ENJOY GOOD MOOD FOOD**

Comforting food can make us feel all kinds of good,
so today enjoy a comfort food that makes you feel good.
Whether you're cooking it yourself or decamping elsewhere
to be cooked for, it's a great opportunity to get together
with friends and family and create a good-mood meal
to share with the people you love. **Jamie**

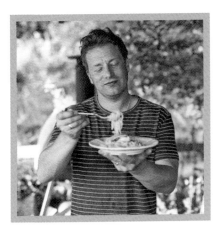

362. **A MEMORY TO CHERISH**

What's a memory you recall and cherish from your early years? Recalling good memories is not only nice, but it's also been proven to boost your overall happiness. So take a trip down memory lane and relive those moments!

363. **NOTICE A DETAIL**

Today, pay attention to a detail in your day. Research shows we tend to be happier when we focus on the activity we're doing, instead of thinking about something else. In fact, paying attention in the moment is a better predictor of happiness than the activity itself! To help you pay attention, try to notice a detail in an everyday activity. When you're out walking or exercising, feel your feet on the ground. While washing the dishes, admire the soap bubbles. Or if you're in a new place, try to find an interesting detail in your surroundings.

364. **PLAN THE YEAR AHEAD**

Although we are almost at the end of this book, it's simply
the beginning of something new. Take a moment and pick
a micro-action or two that you'd like to make into habits
next year. What do you want to achieve? What do you want
to learn? What do you want to improve in yourself?
It's never too early or too late to start!

365. **YOU**

Congratulations! You've reached the final micro-action of this book. Now find a place on your bookshelf where you can store this book to come back to when you need inspiration. Then set yourself a calendar reminder for a month or three from now, when you'll take an hour to just sit down and flip through the pages and reflect.

Thank you for this journey, and keep up being you.

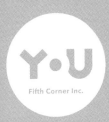

GET MORE MICRO-ACTIONS WITH YOU-APP

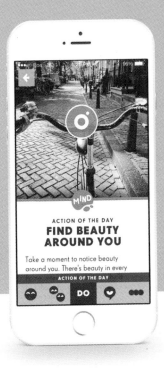

AND JOIN THE WORLD'S MOST POSITIVE COMMUNITY

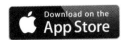
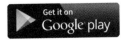

Every day working on the YOU-app we get testimonials from people who have used the app and found micro-actions helpful. People cite being more mindful, more positive, making healthier choices, and understanding the power of small actions. Then at times there are longer, personal stories that just make us stop, and remind us why we do the work we do. This was one of those:

Dear YOU,

When I stumbled across YOU-app in January I was in a bad place in my life. I had lost my way and I was barely existing through each day. I had become a stranger to happiness – something completely unlike the "me" I had always known.

I've found that my joy has come back through the daily actions, but in particular through my Keep It Up actions. I started out with the Read Something New micro-action which broke the monotony of reading for my studies. It reminded me that there is a whole world out there, which is the reason I'm putting myself through the slog of getting a degree at the ripe age of 39.

My next Keep It Up action was to Find Micro-Magic in Your Day. This helped me to find little moments of awe and gratitude each day, which I noticed became underlying awareness of gratitude throughout the day. I moved on to taking "me" time which is so important. I realize that now. The lack of downtime does take its toll. It's not easy as a homeschooling mom, coupled with minimal finances. I sometimes feel guilty, wanting time for myself. It makes me feel like a bad mother some days. But this action energized me and was so valuable. I feel like the dip I went through last year was exactly that. Just a dip. Not an irreversible change. So thank you!

Toni

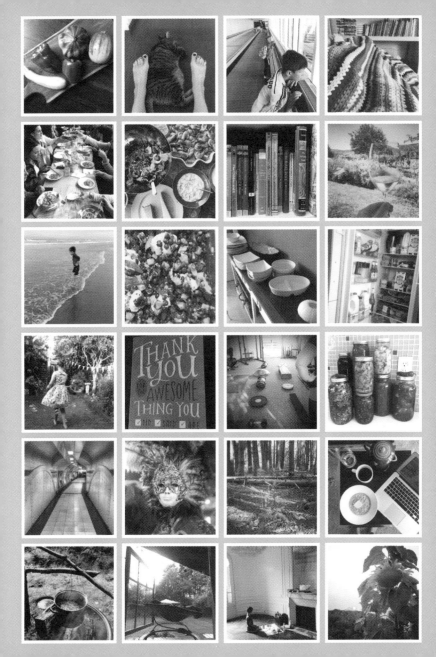

Permissions

With thanks to the following YOU-app users for their contributions:
BeeW, ChrisForestFood, cositas, divadiane, DocBells, GrahamEttridge,
HappyDaysNo.1, InternationalMenu, J_furr, JimmyCSmitz, Leap2itCate,
lindseyevans, livelittleadventures, Mamacha, mariastrat, NikNyg, Picasso, rob7,
spots_of_time, strawberry_girl, supersteph, twintasticand2more

The Experiment, LLC, 220 East 23rd Street, Suite 301, New York, NY 10010-4674
www.theexperimentpublishing.com

This book contains the opinions and ideas of its authors. It is intended to provide helpful and informative material on the subjects addressed in the book. It is sold with the understanding that the authors and publisher are not engaged in rendering medical, health, or any other kind of personal professional services in the book. The authors and publisher specifically disclaim all responsibility for any liability, loss, or risk—personal or otherwise—that is incurred as a consequence, directly or indirectly, of the use and application of any of the contents of this book.

Many of the designations used by manufacturers and sellers to distinguish their products are claimed as trademarks. Where those designations appear in this book and The Experiment was aware of a trademark claim, the designations have been capitalized.

The Experiment's books are available at special discounts when purchased in bulk for premiums and sales promotions as well as for fund-raising or educational use. For details, contact us at info@theexperimentpublishing.com.

Library of Congress Cataloging-in-Publication Data available upon request

ISBN 978-1-61519-380-6
Ebook ISBN 978-1-61519-381-3

Cover design by Sarah Schneider | Text design by Smith & Gilmour

Manufactured in China
Distributed by Workman Publishing Company, Inc.
Distributed simultaneously in Canada by Thomas Allen & Son Ltd.

First printing December 2016
10 9 8 7 6 5 4 3 2 1